Rheumatoid Arthritis Diet Cookbook

100+ Anti-Inflammatory Recipes to Inflammation Relief and Manage Symptoms with 30 Days Meal Plan

Ariah Johnson

Copyright© 2024 by Ariah Johnson

All rights reserved worldwide.

No part of this book may be reproduced or transmitted in any form or by any means, electronic or mechanical, including photo- copying, recording or by any information storage and retrieval system, without written permission from the publisher, except for the inclusion of brief quotations in a review.

Warning-Disclaimer

The purpose of this book is to educate and entertain. The author or publisher does not guarantee that anyone following the techniques, suggestions, tips, ideas, or strategies will become successful. The author and publisher shall have either liability or responsibility to anyone with respect to any loss or damage caused, or alleged to be caused, directly or indirectly by the information contained in this book.

Table of Contents

INTRODUCTION 6
    What is Rheumatoid Arthritis? 7
    What Causes Rheumatoid Arthritis? 7
    Empowered Eating for Rheumatoid Arthritis 8

CHAPTER 1: BREAKFAST 9
    Turmeric and Spinach Scrambled Eggs 9
    Quinoa Breakfast Bowl with Blueberries 10
    Sweet Potato and Avocado Toast 11
    Chia Seed Pudding with Mixed Berries 12
    Green Smoothie with Kale and Pineapple 13
    Avocado and Egg Breakfast Wrap 14
    Coconut Yogurt with Turmeric Granola 15
    Berry Almond Overnight Oats 16
    Sweet Potato and Kale Hash 17
    Spinach and Feta Omelette 18
    Ginger Pear Smoothie Bowl 19
    Almond Butter and Banana Toast 20
    Turmeric Oatmeal with Blueberries 21
    Vegan Banana Pancakes 22
    Egg Muffins with Mushrooms and Spinach 23
    Quinoa and Berry Breakfast Cups of 24
    Zucchini Bread with Walnuts 25
    Almond Butter Toast with Chia Seeds 26

CHAPTER 2: VEGETABLES AND SIDES 27
    Zesty Lemon Broccoli 27
    Cauliflower Tabouleh 28
    Grilled Asparagus with Lemon 29
    Roasted Butternut Squash with Pecans 30
    Garlic Mashed Cauliflower 31
    Sautéed Spinach with Garlic and Lemon 32
    Roasted Sweet Potatoes with Turmeric 33
    Steamed Green Beans with Almonds 34
    Roasted Carrots with Honey and Ginger 35
    Cauliflower Rice with Herbs 36
    Spiced Lentil and Carrot Patties 37
    Kale and Almond Salad 38
    Roasted Beets with Olive Oil and Herbs 39
    Carrot and Apple Slaw 40
    Stuffed Bell Peppers with Quinoa 41
    Roasted Eggplant with Tahini 42

CHAPTER 3: SOUP AND SALAD 43
    Sweet Potato and Ginger Soup 43
    Hearty Lentil Stew 44
    Chicken and Vegetable Soup 45
    Tomato and White Bean Soup 46
    Carrot and Coriander Soup 47

Creamy Butternut Squash Soup 48
Pea and Mint Soup 49
Spicy Black Bean Soup 50
Broccoli and Almond Soup 51
Mushroom and Thyme Stew 52
Mediterranean Chickpea Salad 53
Cucumber and Dill Salad 54
Quinoa and Roasted Beet Salad 55
Tomato and Turmeric Stew 56
Lentil and Spinach Soup 57
Roasted Beet and Goat Cheese Salad 58
Chicken Noodle Soup with Turmeric 59
Vegetable Minestrone 60

CHAPTER 4: FISH AND SEAFOOD **61**
Baked Salmon with Dill and Lemon 61
Grilled Tuna with Avocado Salsa 62
Garlic Shrimp with Zucchini Noodles 63
Broiled Cod with Turmeric and Garlic 64
Seared Scallops with Cauliflower Purée 65
Turmeric Spiced Baked Tilapia 66
Lemon Herb Grilled Mackerel 67
Smoked Salmon and Avocado Salad 68
Pesto-Crusted Halibut 69
Coconut Curry Salmon 70
Fish Tacos with Mango Salsa 71
Pan-Seared Trout with Almonds 72
Shrimp and Broccoli Stir-Fry 73

CHAPTER 5: VEGAN AND VEGETARIAN **74**
Vegan Lentil and Spinach Curry 74
Vegan Stuffed Peppers with Quinoa 75
Eggplant and Lentil Bolognese 76
Spicy Tofu Stir-Fry with Vegetables 77
Butternut Squash Risotto 78
Chickpea and Sweet Potato Stew 79
Zucchini Lasagna with Cashew Cheese 80
Vegan Cauliflower Tacos 81
Quinoa Stuffed Tomatoes 82
Moroccan Vegetable Tagine 83
Vegan Eggplant Parmesan 84
Roasted Vegetable Quinoa Bowl 85
Vegan Vegetable Paella 86

CHAPTER 6: POULTRY AND MEAT **88**
Grilled Chicken with Turmeric and Lime 88
Roasted Chicken with Garlic and Thyme 89
Chicken and Sweet Potato Stir-Fry 90
Lemon Rosemary Roasted Turkey 91
Grilled Chicken Skewers with Veggies 92
Balsamic Glazed Chicken Thighs 93
Chicken and Zucchini Lettuce Wraps 94
Slow-cooked beef and Sweet Potato Stew 95

Grilled Turkey Burgers with Avocado 96
Herb-Crusted Lamb Chops 97
Beef and Barley Soup 98
Chicken Stir-Fry with Bell Peppers 99
Turkey and Zucchini Patties 100
Spiced Turkey and Sweet Potato Hash 101
Ginger Chicken Lettuce Wraps 102
Slow Cooker Chicken and Carrot Stew 103
Grilled Lamb with Mint Sauce 104

CHAPTER 7: SNACKS **105**
Roasted Chickpeas with Paprika 105
Almond Butter and Banana Bites 106
Apple Slices with Almond Butter 106
Baked Sweet Potato Chips 107
Carrot Sticks with Hummus 108
Kale Chips with Sea Salt 108
Cucumber Slices with Guacamole 109
Roasted Pumpkin Seeds 110
Turmeric Spiced Popcorn 111

CHAPTER 8: DESSERTS **112**
Coconut Mango Chia Pudding 112
Avocado Chocolate Mousse 113
Baked Cinnamon Apples with Walnuts 114
Almond Flour Brownies 115
Blueberry Chia Pudding 116
Turmeric Spiced Banana Bread 117
Dark Chocolate Avocado Truffles 118
Almond Butter Chocolate Chip Cookies 119
Lemon Coconut Energy Balls 120
Banana Almond Oat Bars 121

30 DAYS MEAL PLAN **122**

INTRODUCTION

Living with rheumatoid arthritis (RA) may be a difficult journey, characterized by persistent pain, inflammation, and the difficulty of completing daily chores. But what if I told you that one of the most effective weapons for combating this illness is right in your kitchen? The Rheumatoid Arthritis Diet Cookbook provides tasty, nutritious dishes to help you decrease inflammation joint discomfort, and enhance your overall health.

This cookbook is about more than simply food; it is also about gaining control of your health. Using carefully chosen products and simple recipes, you'll discover how the appropriate diet may help reduce RA symptoms. You don't have to sacrifice taste to feel better—this cookbook demonstrates how healthy eating can be both fulfilling and pleasant.

This book contains recipes that have been particularly designed for people with RA. From substantial breakfasts to filling meals and even decadent desserts, each dish contains anti-inflammatory foods and critical nutrients that may help your body recover from the inside. Whether you've just been diagnosed or have been treating RA for years, these meals can help you take a proactive approach to your health.

However, this cookbook is more than simply a compilation of recipes. It's your guide through the difficulties of rheumatoid arthritis, with helpful recommendations on food, lifestyle adjustments, and meal planning. You'll also learn to avoid frequent inflammatory triggers and replace them with healthier options to encourage recovery.

If you want to make a good change in your life and lessen the influence of RA on your daily routine, this book is for you. The recipes in this book are simple yet revolutionary, assisting you in laying the groundwork for a healthy diet that supports your body's battle against inflammation. Begin cooking now, and let this book be the first step in regaining your health, one meal at a time.

What is Rheumatoid Arthritis?

Rheumatoid arthritis, or RA, is a chronic disorder that affects your joints, causing pain, swelling, and stiffness. It occurs when your immune system, which typically defends your body from infection, attacks healthy joint tissues by mistake. This causes inflammation in your joints, making them uncomfortable, swollen, and difficult to move.

RA mostly affects the tiny joints in your hands, wrists, and feet but may extend to other body regions. The soreness and stiffness may be greater in the morning or after resting. If RA is not adequately controlled, it may develop joint deterioration over time, making it difficult to do daily actions such as holding things, walking, or even opening jars.

Unlike other varieties of arthritis caused by aging or injury, rheumatoid arthritis may afflict persons of any age and often begins between the ages of 30 and 60. Women are more likely than males to acquire RA, and the disease may run in families.

While there is no cure for RA, the good news is that you may alleviate symptoms and improve your quality of life with proper treatment and lifestyle modifications, such as a nutritious diet. That's where this cookbook comes in: to help you manage RA by eating meals full of anti-inflammatory ingredients tailored to benefit your health.

What Causes Rheumatoid Arthritis?

The specific etiology of rheumatoid arthritis (RA) is unknown, however, it occurs when the immune system mistakenly attacks healthy joint tissue. Normally, our immune systems defend us from germs and diseases, but with RA, they get confused and produce joint inflammation.

RA may be caused by a variety of reasons, including:

Genetics: If you have a family history of RA, you may be more likely to acquire it. Having a family member with RA, however, does not guarantee that you will get the disease.

Environment: Certain environmental variables, such as smoking or exposure to pollution, may raise your chance of having RA, particularly if you are genetically susceptible to it.

Hormones: Because RA is more frequent in women, experts suspect hormones may play a role in its development.

Infections: Some studies show that, although infections may not directly cause RA, they may cause the immune system to overreact in patients who are already at risk.

Lifestyle Factors: Smoking and being overweight might raise the likelihood of having RA or exacerbate its symptoms.

Empowered Eating for Rheumatoid Arthritis

When you have rheumatoid arthritis (RA), every meal may help your body repair and minimize inflammation. Empowered eating is making conscious food choices that may help alleviate symptoms and enhance overall well-being. The appropriate meals may give your body the nutrition it needs to combat inflammation, relieve joint discomfort, and give you more energy to live your best life.

You can make meals that are both tasty and good for your health by concentrating on full, nutrient-dense foods. Leafy greens, berries, fatty fish, nuts, and seeds are high in antioxidants and good fats, which assist in reducing inflammation and joint discomfort. Simultaneously, eliminating processed meals and adding sweets and bad fats will help prevent flare-ups and maintain your body's balance.

Empowered eating for RA does not include rigorous diets or restrictions. Eating healthy meals that fuel your body and taste good is important. Simple modifications, such as replacing packaged snacks with fresh fruits or more omega-3-rich foods like salmon and walnuts, may significantly impact your feelings.

With the dishes in this cookbook, you'll see that empowered eating can be a fun experience. Each meal is made with your health in mind, combining deliciousness with anti-inflammatory ingredients that benefit your joints and general well-being. Whether it's a colorful salad, a nourishing soup, or a delightful smoothie, each meal may help you feel stronger, more energetic, and more in control of your RA.

CHAPTER 1: BREAKFAST

Turmeric and Spinach Scrambled Eggs

Prep Time: 5 minutes

Cook Time: 10 minutes

Serving: 2

Ingredients

- 4 large eggs
- 1 cup of fresh spinach, chopped
- 1/4 teaspoon ground turmeric
- 1 tablespoon olive oil or avocado oil
- 1/4 cup of unsweetened almond milk (or any plant-based milk)
- Salt and pepper to taste
- 1/4 teaspoon garlic powder (optional)

Instructions

1. Mix the eggs, almond milk, turmeric, garlic powder (if using), salt, and pepper in a medium bowl until thoroughly combined.
2. Heat the olive oil in a nonstick skillet over medium heat.
3. Add the chopped spinach to the pan and cook for 1-2 minutes or until wilted.
4. Pour the egg mixture over the spinach, then use a spatula to scramble the eggs gently. Cook the eggs for 3-4 minutes or until set yet tender.
5. Remove from the heat and serve immediately.

Nutrition Information (Per Serving):

Calories: 180 Protein: 12g Carbohydrates: 3g Fat: 13g Fiber: 1g Sodium: 180mg Sugar: 0g

Quinoa Breakfast Bowl with Blueberries

Prep Time: 5 minutes

Cook Time: 15 minutes

Serving: 2

Ingredients

- 1/2 cup of quinoa, rinsed
- 1 cup of unsweetened almond milk (or any plant-based milk)
- 1/2 teaspoon ground cinnamon
- 1/2 teaspoon vanilla extract
- 1 tablespoon chia seeds
- 1 cup of fresh blueberries
- 2 tablespoons chopped almonds
- 1 tablespoon maple syrup or honey (optional)
- 1/4 cup of unsweetened coconut flakes (optional)

Instructions

1. In a small saucepan, mix the quinoa and almond milk. Bring to a boil over medium heat.
2. Once boiling, decrease the heat to low, cover, and cook for 12-15 minutes or until the quinoa is cooked and the liquid has been absorbed.
3. Mix in the cinnamon, vanilla essence, and chia seeds. Allow the mixture to settle for a minute so that the chia seeds can thicken the texture somewhat.
4. Divide the quinoa mixture into two dishes.
5. Garnish each dish with fresh blueberries, sliced almonds, coconut flakes (if used), and a drizzle of maple syrup or honey for sweetness.
6. Serve warm and enjoy!

Nutrition Information (Per Serving):

Calories: 300 Protein: 8g Carbohydrates: 45gFat: 9g Fiber: 7g Sodium: 40mg Sugar: 10g

Sweet Potato and Avocado Toast

Prep Time: 5 minutes

Cook Time: 10 minutes

Serving: 2

Ingredients

- 1 large sweet potato, sliced into 1/4-inch thick pieces (about 4 slices)
- 1 ripe avocado
- 1 tablespoon olive oil
- 1/4 teaspoon ground turmeric
- 1/4 teaspoon smoked paprika (optional)
- Salt and pepper to taste
- 1 tablespoon lemon juice
- 2 teaspoons chia seeds or hemp seeds (optional)

Instructions

1. Preheat a grill pan or skillet to medium heat. Lightly brush both sides of the sweet potato slices with olive oil.
2. Grill the sweet potato slices in the pan for 5-6 minutes on each side or until slightly brown.
3. While the sweet potato cooks, scoop the avocado into a small bowl. Mash it with a fork, then add the lemon juice, turmeric, salt, pepper, and smoked paprika (if using).
4. When the sweet potato slices are done, place them on a dish.
5. Spread the mashed avocado mixture equally on each sweet potato slice.
6. To provide additional nourishment, sprinkle chia or hemp seeds on top (optional).
7. Serve immediately and enjoy!

Nutrition Information (Per Serving):

Calories: 220 Protein: 3g Carbohydrates: 23g Fat: 15g Fiber: 7g Sodium: 100mg Sugar: 4g

Chia Seed Pudding with Mixed Berries

Prep Time: 5 minutes

Chill Time: 4 hours or overnight

Serving: 2

Ingredients

- 1/4 cup of chia seeds
- 1 cup of unsweetened almond milk (or any plant-based milk)
- 1 tablespoon maple syrup or honey (optional)
- 1/2 teaspoon vanilla extract
- 1/2 cup of mixed berries (blueberries, strawberries, raspberries)
- 1 tablespoon slivered almonds (optional)
- Fresh mint leaves for garnish (optional)

Instructions

1. In a medium mixing bowl, combine the almond milk, chia seeds, maple syrup (if using), and vanilla extract.
2. Stir well to ensure that the chia seeds are uniformly dispersed. Allow it to settle for approximately 5 minutes before stirring again to break up clumps.
3. Cover the bowl and refrigerate for at least 4 hours, ideally overnight, until the pudding reaches your preferred consistency.
4. When ready to serve, split the chia seed pudding into two dishes or glasses.
5. Top each plate with mixed berries and a sprinkling of slivered almonds for crunch. Garnish with fresh mint leaves if preferred.
6. Serve cold, and enjoy!

Nutrition Information (Per Serving):

Calories: 200 Protein: 5g Carbohydrates: 20g Fat: 10g Fiber: 10g Sodium: 60mg Sugar: 8g

Green Smoothie with Kale and Pineapple

Prep Time: 5 minutes

Serving: 2

Ingredients

- 1 cup of fresh kale, chopped and stems removed
- 1 cup of fresh pineapple chunks
- 1 ripe banana
- 1/2 cup of unsweetened almond milk (or any plant-based milk)
- 1/2 cup of water
- 1 tablespoon chia seeds
- 1 tablespoon fresh lemon juice
- 1/2 teaspoon fresh ginger, grated (optional)
- Ice cubes (optional)

Instructions

1. Add the kale, pineapple, banana, almond milk, water, chia seeds, lemon juice, and ginger (if using) to a blender.
2. Blend at high speeds until smooth and creamy. Add some ice cubes and mix again if you want a cooler smoothie.
3. Taste and adjust for sweetness or tartness by adding extra pineapple or lemon juice as required.
4. Pour the smoothie into two glasses and serve immediately.

Nutrition Information (Per Serving):

Calories: 150 Protein: 3g Carbohydrates: 34g Fat: 3g Fiber: 6g Sodium: 60mg Sugar: 18g

Avocado and Egg Breakfast Wrap

Prep Time: 5 minutes

Cook Time: 10 minutes

Serving: 2

Ingredients

- 2 large eggs
- 1 ripe avocado
- 2 whole wheat or gluten-free wraps
- 1/2 cup of fresh spinach, chopped
- 1 tablespoon olive oil or avocado oil
- 1/4 teaspoon ground turmeric
- 1/4 teaspoon garlic powder (optional)
- Salt and pepper to taste
- 1 tablespoon fresh cilantro or parsley, chopped (optional)
- 1 tablespoon lemon juice

Instructions

1. In a small mixing bowl, combine the avocado, lemon juice, garlic powder (if using), salt, and pepper. Set aside.
2. Heat the olive oil in a nonstick skillet over medium heat. Crack the eggs into a pan and season with turmeric, salt, and pepper.
3. Cook the eggs gently until totally set, approximately 3-4 minutes.
4. Warm the wraps in a different skillet or microwave for a few seconds to make them more malleable.
5. Spread the mashed avocado equally on each wrap. Combine the chopped spinach and scrambled eggs.
6. Sprinkle with fresh cilantro or parsley, if desired.
7. Fold the sides of the wrap inwards and roll securely. Cut in half and serve immediately.

Nutrition Information (Per Serving):

Calories: 320 Protein: 12g Carbohydrates: 28g Fat: 20g Fiber: 8g Sodium: 260mg Sugar: 1g

Coconut Yogurt with Turmeric Granola

Prep Time: 5 minutes

Cook Time: 20 minutes (for granola)

Serving: 2

Ingredients

- For the Turmeric Granola:
- 1 cup of rolled oats (gluten-free if needed)
- 1/4 cup of almonds, chopped
- 2 tablespoons chia seeds
- 1/4 teaspoon ground turmeric
- 1/4 teaspoon ground cinnamon
- 2 tablespoons coconut oil, melted
- 2 tablespoons maple syrup or honey
- For the Yogurt Bowl:
- 1 cup of coconut yogurt (unsweetened)
- 1/2 cup of fresh berries (blueberries, raspberries, or strawberries)
- 2 tablespoons shredded coconut (optional)
- 1 tablespoon chia seeds or flaxseeds (optional)

Instructions

1. Preheat the oven to 325°F (160°C), and line a baking sheet with parchment paper.
2. Combine the rolled oats, chopped almonds, chia seeds, turmeric, and cinnamon in a large mixing bowl.
3. In a small dish, combine the melted coconut oil and maple syrup. Pour the mixture over the oats, stirring until uniformly covered.
4. Spread the granola mixture in an equal layer on the prepared baking sheet.
5. Bake for 15-20 minutes, stirring halfway through, or until golden and crisp. Allow it to cool fully.
6. Divide the coconut yogurt into two dishes. Top each bowl with a couple of tablespoons of turmeric granola, fresh berries, and shredded coconut (if desired).
7. For additional nourishment, sprinkle chia or flax seeds on top.
8. Serve immediately and enjoy!

Nutrition Information (Per Serving):

Calories: 350 Protein: 7g Carbohydrates: 35g Fat: 18g Fiber: 9g Sodium: 30mg Sugar: 12g

Berry Almond Overnight Oats

Prep Time: 5 minutes

Chill Time: 4 hours or overnight

Serving: 2

Ingredients

- 1 cup of rolled oats (gluten-free if needed)
- 1 cup of unsweetened almond milk (or any plant-based milk)
- 1/2 cup of fresh mixed berries
- 2 tablespoons almond butter
- 1 tablespoon chia seeds
- 1/2 teaspoon vanilla extract
- 1 tablespoon maple syrup or honey (optional)
- 2 tablespoons sliced almonds
- 1/2 teaspoon ground cinnamon (optional)

Instructions

1. Mix the rolled oats, almond milk, chia seeds, vanilla essence, and maple syrup (if desired). Stir well to mix.
2. Add half of the mixed berries to the oat mixture and stir gently.
3. Cover the dish or jar and chill for at least 4 hours or overnight to let the oats and chia seeds absorb the liquid.
4. In the morning, mix the oats well. If you desire a thinner consistency, use additional almond milk.
5. Divide the overnight oatmeal into two dishes or jars. Top each plate with the leftover mixed berries, a drizzle of almond butter, sliced almonds, and optional cinnamon.
6. Serve cold, and enjoy!

Nutrition Information (Per Serving):

Calories: 320 Protein: 9g Carbohydrates: 40g Fat: 14g Fiber: 9g Sodium: 50mg Sugar: 10g

Sweet Potato and Kale Hash

Prep Time: 10 minutes

Cook Time: 20 minutes

Serving: 2

Ingredients

- 1 large sweet potato, peeled and diced into small cubes
- 1 cup of fresh kale, chopped and stems removed
- 1 small onion, diced
- 1 tablespoon olive oil or avocado oil
- 1/2 teaspoon ground turmeric
- 1/2 teaspoon smoked paprika
- Salt and pepper to taste
- 1/4 teaspoon garlic powder (optional)
- 2 large eggs (optional for added protein)
- Fresh parsley or cilantro for garnish (optional)

Instructions

1. Heat the olive oil in a large pan over medium heat.
2. Add the diced sweet potatoes and onions to the skillet. Season with turmeric, smoked paprika, garlic powder (optional), salt, and pepper.
3. Cook, stirring periodically, for 10-12 minutes or until the sweet potatoes soften and brown.
4. Cook for 5-7 minutes, stirring periodically, until the kale has wilted and the sweet potatoes are cooked.
5. If you add eggs, make little wells in the hash and break one into each. Cover the pan and simmer for another 3-4 minutes or until the eggs are done to your preference.
6. Remove from the heat and garnish with fresh parsley or cilantro, if preferred.
7. Serve hot, and enjoy!

Nutrition Information (Per Serving):

Calories: 250 (without eggs) Carbohydrates: 35gFat: 10g Fiber: 7g Sodium: 120mg Sugar: 7g

Spinach and Feta Omelette

Prep Time: 5 minutes

Cook Time: 10 minutes

Serving: 2

Ingredients

- 4 large eggs
- 1/2 cup of fresh spinach, chopped
- 1/4 cup of crumbled feta cheese
- 1 tablespoon olive oil or avocado oil
- Salt and pepper to taste
- 1/4 teaspoon garlic powder (optional)
- 1 tablespoon fresh parsley or dill, chopped (optional)

Instructions

1. In a medium bowl, whisk together the eggs, salt, pepper, and garlic powder (if using) until thoroughly blended.
2. Heat the olive oil in a nonstick skillet over medium heat.
3. Add the chopped spinach to the pan and cook for 1-2 minutes or until wilted.
4. Pour the egg mixture over the spinach and heat for 3-4 minutes or until the edges firm.
5. Sprinkle the crumbled feta cheese evenly over the eggs.
6. Fold the omelet in half and cook for 2-3 minutes until the eggs are completely set and the cheese is melted.
7. Remove from the heat and garnish with fresh parsley or dill, if preferred.
8. Serve immediately and enjoy!

Nutrition Information (Per Serving):

Calories: 230 Protein: 14g Carbohydrates: 2g Fat: 18g Fiber: 1g Sodium: 320mg Sugar: 1g

Ginger Pear Smoothie Bowl

Prep Time: 5 minutes

Serving: 2

Ingredients

- 1 ripe pear, cored and chopped
- 1/2 cup of unsweetened almond milk
- 1/2 cup of plain coconut yogurt (unsweetened)
- 1 tablespoon fresh ginger, grated
- 1/2 frozen banana
- 1 tablespoon chia seeds
- 1/4 teaspoon ground cinnamon
- 1 teaspoon honey or maple syrup (optional)
- Ice cubes (optional for a thicker texture)
- Toppings:
- 1/4 cup of granola
- 1 tablespoon pumpkin seeds
- 1/4 cup of fresh berries (optional)
- 1 tablespoon shredded coconut (optional)

Instructions

1. Blend the diced pear, almond milk, coconut yogurt, grated ginger, frozen banana, chia seeds, cinnamon, and honey (if using).
2. Blend until smooth and creamy. If you like a thicker texture, add a few ice cubes.
3. Pour the smoothie into two bowls.
4. Top each bowl with granola, pumpkin seeds, fresh berries, shredded coconut, or any other toppings you choose.
5. Serve immediately and enjoy!

Nutrition Information (Per Serving):

Calories: 260 Protein: 6g Carbohydrates: 40g Fat: 10g Fiber: 8g Sodium: 50mg Sugar: 20g

Almond Butter and Banana Toast

Prep Time: 5 minutes

Serving: 2

Ingredients

- 2 slices whole grain or gluten-free bread
- 2 tablespoons almond butter
- 1 ripe banana, sliced
- 1 teaspoon chia seeds or flaxseeds (optional)
- 1/4 teaspoon ground cinnamon (optional)
- 1 teaspoon honey or maple syrup (optional)

Instructions

1. Toast the bread pieces in a toaster or a skillet until golden and crispy.
2. Spread 1 tablespoon of almond butter onto each piece of bread.
3. Top each slice with banana slices, putting them equally on the almond butter.
4. For added taste and nutrients, sprinkle chia or flax seeds and a splash of cinnamon on top. If you want to add sweetness, drizzle with honey or maple syrup (optional).
5. Serve immediately and enjoy!

Nutrition Information (Per Serving):

Calories: 300 Protein: 8g Carbohydrates: 34g Fat: 16g Fiber: 7g Sodium: 160mg Sugar: 10g

Turmeric Oatmeal with Blueberries

Prep Time: 5 minutes

Cook Time: 10 minutes

Serving: 2

Ingredients

- 1 cup of rolled oats (gluten-free if needed)
- 2 cups of unsweetened almond milk (or any plant-based milk)
- 1/2 teaspoon ground turmeric
- 1/4 teaspoon ground cinnamon
- 1 tablespoon chia seeds
- 1 tablespoon maple syrup or honey (optional)
- 1/2 cup of fresh blueberries
- 1 tablespoon slivered almonds or walnuts (optional)
- 1 teaspoon vanilla extract (optional)

Instructions

1. Mix the oats, almond milk, turmeric, cinnamon, and chia seeds in a medium saucepan. Stir thoroughly.
2. Bring to a moderate boil over medium heat, then lower to a low heat and simmer for 5-7 minutes, stirring regularly, until the oats have softened and absorbed most of the liquid.
3. Mix in the maple syrup and vanilla extract (if using).
4. Divide the oatmeal into two dishes. Top each dish with fresh blueberries, slivered almonds or walnuts, and an additional sprinkling of cinnamon, if preferred.
5. Serve warm and enjoy!

Nutrition Information (Per Serving):

Calories: 280 Protein: 8g Carbohydrates: 45g Fat: 8g Fiber: 9g Sodium: 60mgSugar: 12g

Vegan Banana Pancakes

Prep Time: 5 minutes

Cook Time: 10 minutes

Serving: 2

Ingredients

- 1 ripe banana, mashed
- 1 cup of whole wheat flour (or gluten-free flour)
- 1 tablespoon chia seeds or flaxseeds
- 1/2 teaspoon baking powder
- 1/4 teaspoon ground cinnamon
- 1 teaspoon vanilla extract
- 1 tablespoon maple syrup (optional)
- 1 cup of unsweetened almond milk (or any plant-based milk)
- 1 tablespoon coconut oil (for cooking)
- Fresh fruit, nuts, or syrup for topping (optional)

Instructions

1. Mix the chia seeds or flaxseeds in a small bowl with 3 tablespoons of water. Allow it to settle for 5 minutes to get a gel-like consistency (this will be your egg replacement).
2. In a mixing bowl, mash the ripe banana. Whisk in the chia or flaxseed combination, almond milk, vanilla extract, and maple syrup (if using) until combined.
3. In a separate bowl, combine flour, baking powder, and cinnamon.
4. Combine the dry ingredients with the wet mixture and whisk until just mixed. Take care not to over mix.
5. Heat a nonstick skillet or griddle over medium heat, then coat with coconut oil.
6. Pour roughly 1/4 cup of pancake batter into the skillet for each pancake. Cook for 2-3 minutes until bubbles appear on the top, then turn and cook for an additional 2-3 minutes until golden brown.
7. Repeat with the remaining batter, adding extra oil to the skillet if necessary.
8. Serve warm pancakes topped with fresh fruit, nuts, or syrup.

Nutrition Information (Per Serving):

Calories: 280 Protein: 6g Carbohydrates: 45g Fat: 9g Fiber: 7g Sodium: 180mg Sugar: 10g

Egg Muffins with Mushrooms and Spinach

Prep Time: 10 minutes

Cook Time: 20 minutes

Serving: 6 (makes 12 muffins)

Ingredients

- 6 large eggs
- 1/2 cup of fresh spinach, chopped
- 1/2 cup of mushrooms, diced
- 1/4 cup of onions, finely chopped
- 1/4 cup of almond milk (or any plant-based milk)
- 1/4 teaspoon garlic powder (optional)
- Salt and pepper to taste
- 1 tablespoon olive oil or avocado oil (for sautéing)
- 1/4 cup of feta cheese, crumbled (optional)

Instructions

1. Preheat the oven to 350°F/175°C and gently butter a 12-cup muffin pan.
2. Heat the olive oil in a pan over medium heat. Sauté the onions and mushrooms for 5-7 minutes, until tender and golden. Add the chopped spinach and simmer for 1-2 minutes or until wilted. Remove from heat.
3. In a large mixing bowl, combine the eggs, almond milk, garlic powder (if desired), salt, and pepper.
4. Combine the sautéed mushroom, spinach, and onion combination with the eggs.
5. If using feta cheese, combine it with the egg mixture.
6. Pour the batter equally into the prepared muffin cups, filling them approximately 3/4 full.
7. Bake the egg muffins in a preheated oven for 18-20 minutes or until completely set and faintly browned on top.
8. Let the muffins cool for a few minutes before removing from the pan. Serve warm.

Nutrition Information (Per Serving - 2 muffins):

Calories: 120 Protein: 9g Carbohydrates: 3g Fat: 8g Fiber: 1g Sodium: 150mg Sugar: 1g

Quinoa and Berry Breakfast Cups of

Prep Time: 10 minutes

Cook Time: 15 minutes

Serving: 4

Ingredients

- 1 cup of cooked quinoa
- 1/2 cup of unsweetened almond milk (or any plant-based milk)
- 1 tablespoon maple syrup or honey (optional)
- 1/2 teaspoon vanilla extract
- 1/2 teaspoon ground cinnamon
- 1 cup of fresh mixed berries
- 2 tablespoons chia seeds
- 1/4 cup of slivered almonds (optional)
- 1 tablespoon shredded coconut (optional)

Instructions

1. Mix the cooked quinoa, almond milk, maple syrup, vanilla essence, and cinnamon in a medium saucepan. Cook for 5 minutes over medium heat, stirring periodically, until the mixture is warm and creamy.
2. Remove from heat and add the chia seeds.
3. Divide the quinoa mixture across four dishes or glasses.
4. Top each dish with mixed fresh berries, slivered almonds, and shredded coconut if preferred.
5. Serve warm or cold, according to your liking.

Nutrition Information (Per Serving):

Calories: 210 Protein: 6g Carbohydrates: 30g Fat: 7g Fiber: 6g Sodium: 40mg Sugar: 10g

Zucchini Bread with Walnuts

Prep Time: 15 minutes **Cook Time:** 50-60 minutes **Serving: 8**

Ingredients

- 1 1/2 cups of whole wheat flour (or gluten-free flour)
- 1 teaspoon baking soda
- 1/2 teaspoon baking powder
- 1 teaspoon ground cinnamon
- 1/4 teaspoon ground nutmeg
- 1/4 teaspoon salt
- 1/3 cup of maple syrup or honey
- 1/4 cup of coconut oil, melted
- 2 large eggs (or flax eggs for a vegan option)
- 1 teaspoon vanilla extract
- 1 1/2 cups of zucchini, grated and excess moisture removed
- 1/2 cup of walnuts, chopped
- 1/4 cup of unsweetened applesauce (optional for added moisture)

Instructions

1. Preheat the oven to 350°F (175°C). Grease a 9x5-inch loaf pan.
2. Combine the flour, baking soda, baking powder, cinnamon, nutmeg, and salt in a larger bowl.
3. Mix the eggs (or flax eggs), maple syrup, coconut oil, vanilla extract, and applesauce in a separate large bowl.
4. Gradually incorporate the dry ingredients into the wet until just mixed. Take care not to over mix.
5. Gently incorporate the grated zucchini and chopped walnuts.
6. Pour the batter into the prepared loaf pan and distribute evenly.
7. Bake for 50–60 minutes, or until a toothpick inserted in the middle comes out clean.
8. Let the zucchini bread sit in the pan for 10 minutes before transferring it to a wire rack to cool fully.
9. Slice and serve. Keep leftovers in an airtight jar for up to four days.

Nutrition Information (Per Serving):

Calories: 210 Protein: 5g Carbohydrates: 27g Fat: 10g Fiber: 3g Sodium: 180mg Sugar: 10g

Almond Butter Toast with Chia Seeds

Prep Time: 5 minutes

Serving: 2

Ingredients

- 2 slices whole grain or gluten-free bread
- 2 tablespoons almond butter
- 1 tablespoon chia seeds
- 1 teaspoon honey or maple syrup (optional)
- 1/4 teaspoon ground cinnamon (optional)
- Fresh fruit like banana slices or berries (optional)

Instructions

1. Toast the bread pieces until they're brown and crispy.
2. Spread 1 tablespoon of almond butter onto each piece of bread.
3. Sprinkle the chia seeds evenly over the almond butter.
4. Drizzle honey or maple syrup over top, if desired, then sprinkle with cinnamon for added taste.
5. Optionally, top with fresh banana slices or berries for an extra nutritional boost.
6. Serve immediately and enjoy!

Nutrition Information (Per Serving):

Calories: 300 Protein: 8g Carbohydrates: 30g Fat: 18g Fiber: 8g Sodium: 150mg Sugar: 5g

CHAPTER 2: VEGETABLES AND SIDES

Zesty Lemon Broccoli

Prep Time: 5 minutes

Cook Time: 10 minutes

Serving: 4

Ingredients

- 1 large head of broccoli, cut into florets
- 2 tablespoons olive oil
- 1 garlic clove, minced
- 1 tablespoon lemon zest
- 2 tablespoons fresh lemon juice
- Salt and pepper to taste
- 1/4 teaspoon red pepper flakes (optional)
- 1 tablespoon fresh parsley, chopped (optional)

Instructions

1. Heat a large saucepan of water to a boil. Cook the broccoli florets for 3-4 minutes until cooked yet crisp.
2. Drain the broccoli and put it aside.
3. In a large skillet, heat the olive oil over medium heat. Sauté the minced garlic for 1-2 minutes, until aromatic, taking care not to burn it.
4. Toss the broccoli florets in the pan until coated with garlic and olive oil.
5. Add the lemon zest, juice, salt, pepper, and red pepper flakes (if using). Toss everything together and cook for 2-3 minutes until cooked through.
6. Remove from heat, and if preferred, garnish with fresh parsley.
7. Serve warm and enjoy!

Nutrition Information (Per Serving):

Calories: 90 Protein: 3g Carbohydrates: 9g Fat: 6g Fiber: 4g Sodium: 80mg Sugar: 2g

Cauliflower Tabouleh

Prep Time: 15 minutes

Serving: 4

Ingredients

- 1 medium head of cauliflower, grated or pulsed in a food processor to resemble rice
- 1 cup of fresh parsley, finely chopped
- 1/2 cup of fresh mint leaves, finely chopped
- 1 cup of cucumber, diced
- 1/2 cup of cherry tomatoes, halved
- 1/4 cup of red onion, finely diced
- 1/4 cup of olive oil
- 2 tablespoons fresh lemon juice
- 1 teaspoon lemon zest
- Salt and pepper to taste
- 1/4 teaspoon ground cumin (optional)

Instructions

1. Put the grated cauliflower in a large mixing bowl.
2. Toss the cauliflower, parsley, mint, cucumber, cherry tomatoes, and red onion.
3. In a small mixing bowl, combine the olive oil, lemon juice, zest, salt, pepper, and cumin (if using).
4. Pour the dressing over the cauliflower mixture and toss to coat evenly.
5. Taste and adjust the seasoning as required.
6. Serve immediately or chill for an hour to let the flavors mingle. Garnish with more fresh herbs if desired.

Nutrition Information (Per Serving):

Calories: 130 Protein: 3g Carbohydrates: 10g Fat: 9g Fiber: 4g Sodium: 80mg Sugar: 3g

Grilled Asparagus with Lemon

Prep Time: 5 minutes

Cook Time: 8-10 minutes

Serving: 4

Ingredients

- 1 bunch asparagus, trimmed
- 2 tablespoons olive oil
- 1 tablespoon fresh lemon juice
- 1 teaspoon lemon zest
- Salt and pepper to taste
- 1/4 teaspoon garlic powder (optional)
- 1 tablespoon fresh parsley, chopped (optional)
- Lemon wedges for serving

Instructions

1. Preheat your grill to medium-high (or use a grill pan on the stove).
2. In a small mixing bowl, combine the olive oil, lemon juice, zest, garlic powder (if using), salt, and pepper.
3. Toss the asparagus spears in the lemon and olive oil mixture until completely coated.
4. Place the asparagus on the grill for 4-5 minutes on each side until tender and slightly browned.
5. Remove off the grill and place on a serving platter. Garnish with fresh parsley and serve with additional lemon wedges on the side to squeeze.
6. Serve warm and enjoy!

Nutrition Information (Per Serving):

Calories: 80 Protein: 2g Carbohydrates: 5g Fat: 7g Fiber: 2g Sodium: 50mg Sugar: 2g

Roasted Butternut Squash with Pecans

Prep Time: 10 minutes

Cook Time: 30-35 minutes

Serving: 4

Ingredients

- 1 large butternut squash, peeled, seeded, and cut into 1-inch cubes
- 2 tablespoons olive oil or coconut oil, melted
- 1/2 teaspoon ground cinnamon
- 1/4 teaspoon ground nutmeg
- Salt and pepper to taste
- 1/4 cup of pecans, roughly chopped
- 1 tablespoon maple syrup or honey (optional)
- 1 tablespoon fresh parsley, chopped (optional)

Instructions

1. Preheat the oven to 400 degrees Fahrenheit (200 degrees Celsius) and line a baking sheet with parchment paper.
2. Combine the butternut squash cubes, olive oil, cinnamon, nutmeg, salt, and pepper in a large mixing bowl.
3. Spread the squash equally in a single layer on the prepared baking sheet.
4. Roast in the oven for 25-30 minutes, stirring halfway through or until the squash is soft and caramelized around the edges.
5. Sprinkle the chopped pecans over the squash in the final 5 minutes of roasting, and continue to roast until gently browned.
6. Remove from the oven and, if preferred, sprinkle with maple syrup or honey for extra sweetness.
7. Garnish with fresh parsley and serve warm.

Nutrition Information (Per Serving):

Calories: 180 Protein: 2g Carbohydrates: 24g Fat: 9g Fiber: 4g Sodium: 100mg Sugar: 6g

Garlic Mashed Cauliflower

Prep Time: 10 minutes

Cook Time: 15 minutes

Serving: 4

Ingredients

- 1 large head of cauliflower, cut into florets
- 3 garlic cloves, minced
- 2 tablespoons olive oil or butter (or plant-based butter)
- 1/4 cup of unsweetened almond milk (or any plant-based milk)
- Salt and pepper to taste
- 1 tablespoon fresh parsley, chopped (optional)

Instructions

1. Heat a large saucepan of salted water to a boil. Add the cauliflower florets and simmer for 10-12 minutes or until soft.
2. Drain and put the cauliflower aside.
3. In the same saucepan, heat the olive oil over medium heat. Sauté the minced garlic for 1-2 minutes, until aromatic but not browned.
4. Return the cooked cauliflower to the saucepan and mash with a potato masher or a food processor to get a smoother texture.
5. Add the almond milk and season with salt and pepper to suit. Continue to mash and blend until smooth and creamy.
6. Transfer to a serving dish and top with fresh parsley, if preferred.
7. Serve warm and enjoy!

Nutrition Information (Per Serving):

Calories: 110 Protein: 3g Carbohydrates: 9g Fat: 8g Fiber: 4g Sodium: 90mg Sugar: 3g

Sautéed Spinach with Garlic and Lemon

Prep Time: 5 minutes

Cook Time: 5 minutes

Serving: 4

Ingredients

- 1 tablespoon olive oil
- 3 garlic cloves, minced
- 10 ounces fresh spinach
- 1 tablespoon fresh lemon juice
- Salt and pepper to taste
- Lemon zest for garnish (optional)
- 1 tablespoon fresh parsley, chopped (optional)

Instructions

1. Heat the olive oil in a large pan over medium heat.
2. Sauté the minced garlic for 1-2 minutes, until fragrant, taking care not to burn it.
3. Stir in the fresh spinach and cook until wilted, approximately 2-3 minutes.
4. Once the spinach has wilted, add the lemon juice, salt, and pepper to taste.
5. Remove from heat and place in a serving dish. Garnish with lemon zest and fresh parsley if preferred.
6. Serve immediately and enjoy!

Nutrition Information (Per Serving):

Calories: 70 Protein: 2g Carbohydrates: 3g Fat: 6g Fiber: 2g Sodium: 60mg Sugar: 1g

Roasted Sweet Potatoes with Turmeric

Prep Time: 10 minutes

Cook Time: 30-35 minutes

Serving: 4

Ingredients

- 2 large sweet potatoes, peeled and cut into 1-inch cubes
- 2 tablespoons olive oil or coconut oil, melted
- 1 teaspoon ground turmeric
- 1/2 teaspoon ground cumin
- 1/4 teaspoon smoked paprika (optional)
- Salt and pepper to taste
- Fresh parsley, chopped (for garnish, optional)

Instructions

1. Preheat the oven to 400 degrees Fahrenheit (200 degrees Celsius) and line a baking sheet with parchment paper.
2. In a large mixing bowl, combine the sweet potato cubes, olive oil, turmeric, cumin, smoked paprika (if using), salt, and pepper until equally coated.
3. Spread the sweet potatoes in a single layer on the prepared baking sheet.
4. Roast the sweet potatoes in the oven for 30-35 minutes, tossing halfway through, until soft and caramelized around the edges.
5. Remove from the oven and sprinkle with fresh parsley, if preferred.
6. Serve warm and enjoy!

Nutrition Information (Per Serving):

Calories: 180 Protein: 2g Carbohydrates: 28g Fat: 7g Fiber: 5g Sodium: 140mg Sugar: 7g

Steamed Green Beans with Almonds

Prep Time: 5 minutes

Cook Time: 10 minutes

Serving: 4

Ingredients

- 1 pound fresh green beans, trimmed
- 2 tablespoons olive oil
- 1/4 cup of sliced almonds, toasted
- 1 garlic clove, minced
- 1 tablespoon fresh lemon juice
- Salt and pepper to taste
- 1 tablespoon fresh parsley, chopped (optional)

Instructions

1. Steam the green beans in a steamer basket over boiling water for 5-7 minutes or until soft yet crisp.
2. While the green beans are steaming, cook the sliced almonds in a dry pan over medium heat, turning regularly, until golden brown. Set aside.
3. In a large skillet, heat the olive oil over medium heat. Sauté the minced garlic for 1-2 minutes, until aromatic.
4. Toss the steamed green beans in the pan with the garlic and olive oil until well coated.
5. Add the fresh lemon juice and season with salt and pepper to taste.
6. Transfer the green beans to a serving plate and garnish with toasted almonds. Garnish with fresh parsley if preferred.
7. Serve warm and enjoy!

Nutrition Information (Per Serving):

Calories: 120 Protein: 3g Carbohydrates: 8g Fat: 9g Fiber: 4g Sodium: 60mg Sugar: 3g

Roasted Carrots with Honey and Ginger

Prep Time: 10 minutes

Cook Time: 25-30 minutes

Serving: 4

Ingredients

- 1 pound carrots, peeled and cut into sticks
- 2 tablespoons olive oil or coconut oil, melted
- 1 tablespoon honey
- 1 tablespoon fresh ginger, grated
- 1/2 teaspoon ground cinnamon (optional)
- Salt and pepper to taste
- 1 tablespoon fresh parsley, chopped (optional)

Instructions

1. Preheat the oven to 400 degrees Fahrenheit (200 degrees Celsius) and line a baking sheet with parchment paper.
2. In a large mixing bowl, combine the carrot sticks, olive oil, honey, grated ginger, cinnamon (if using), salt, and pepper.
3. Place the carrots in a single layer on the prepared baking sheet.
4. Roast the carrots in a warm oven for 25-30 minutes, turning halfway through, until soft and caramelized.
5. Remove from the oven and sprinkle with fresh parsley, if preferred.
6. Serve warm and enjoy!

Nutrition Information (Per Serving):

Calories: 140 Protein: 1g Carbohydrates: 16g Fat: 7g Fiber: 4g Sodium: 100mg Sugar: 9g

Cauliflower Rice with Herbs

Prep Time: 10 minutes

Cook Time: 10 minutes

Serving: 4

Ingredients

- 1 large head of cauliflower, grated or pulsed in a food processor to resemble rice
- 2 tablespoons olive oil
- 1 garlic clove, minced
- 1/4 cup of fresh parsley, chopped
- 2 tablespoons fresh cilantro or dill, chopped
- 1 tablespoon fresh lemon juice
- Salt and pepper to taste
- 1/4 teaspoon ground cumin (optional)

Instructions

1. Heat the olive oil in a large pan over medium heat.
2. Sauté the minced garlic for 1-2 minutes, until fragrant.
3. Cook the cauliflower rice in the pan, turning regularly, until soft but not mushy, about 5-7 minutes.
4. Combine the fresh parsley, cilantro or dill, lemon juice, cumin (if using), salt, and pepper. Mix well to mix.
5. Remove from the fire and adjust seasoning as required.
6. Serve warm and enjoy!

Nutrition Information (Per Serving):

Calories: 90 Protein: 2g Carbohydrates: 7g Fat: 7g Fiber: 3g Sodium: 50mg Sugar: 2g

Spiced Lentil and Carrot Patties

Prep Time: 15 minutes

Cook Time: 25 minutes

Serving: 4 (makes 8 patties)

Ingredients

- 1 cup of cooked lentils (green or brown)
- 1 cup of grated carrots
- 1/4 cup of breadcrumbs (gluten-free if needed)
- 1/4 cup of rolled oats
- 1/4 cup of fresh parsley, chopped
- 1 garlic clove, minced
- 1 tablespoon ground flaxseed (optional)
- 1 teaspoon ground cumin
- 1/2 teaspoon ground coriander
- 1/4 teaspoon smoked paprika
- 1/4 teaspoon ground turmeric
- Salt and pepper to taste
- 2 tablespoons olive oil (for frying)

Instructions

1. Mix the cooked lentils, grated carrots, breadcrumbs, rolled oats, parsley, chopped garlic, and crushed flaxseed in a large mixing bowl.
2. Combine cumin, coriander, smoked paprika, turmeric, salt, and pepper. Mix until everything is fully combined and has a dough-like texture. If the mixture is too dry, add a tablespoon of water; if it is too moist, add more breadcrumbs or oats.
3. Form the mixture into 8 patties approximately 1/2 inch thick.
4. Heat the olive oil in a large pan over medium heat. Fry the patties in batches, 3-4 minutes each side, until golden brown and crisp.
5. Transfer the cooked patties to a dish lined with paper towels to drain any leftover oil.
6. Serve warm, topped with your favorite sauce, or wrapped in greens.

Nutrition Information (Per Serving - 2 patties):

Calories: 180 Protein: 7g Carbohydrates: 23g Fat: 6g Fiber: 7g Sodium: 150mg Sugar: 2g

Kale and Almond Salad

Prep Time: 10 minutes

Serving: 4

Ingredients

- 4 cups of kale, chopped and stems removed
- 1/4 cup of sliced almonds, toasted
- 1/4 cup of dried cranberries (optional)
- 2 tablespoons olive oil
- 1 tablespoon fresh lemon juice
- 1 teaspoon honey or maple syrup
- 1/2 teaspoon Dijon mustard
- Salt and pepper to taste
- 1 tablespoon fresh parsley, chopped (optional)

Instructions

1. Put the chopped kale in a large bowl. Drizzle 1 tablespoon olive oil over the kale and gently massage the leaves with your hands for 1-2 minutes until delicate and supple.
2. In a small mixing bowl, combine the remaining olive oil, lemon juice, honey or maple syrup, Dijon mustard, salt, and pepper to make the dressing.
3. Toss the kale with the dressing until evenly coated.
4. Toss in the roasted almonds and dried cranberries to finish the salad.
5. Garnish with fresh parsley if preferred, and serve immediately.

Nutrition Information (Per Serving):

Calories: 160 Protein: 4g Carbohydrates: 13g Fat: 11g Fiber: 4g Sodium: 70mg Sugar: 6g

Roasted Beets with Olive Oil and Herbs

Prep Time: 10 minutes

Cook Time: 40-45 minutes

Serving: 4

Ingredients

- 4 medium beets, peeled and cut into wedges
- 2 tablespoons olive oil
- 1 teaspoon fresh thyme leaves (or 1/2 teaspoon dried thyme)
- 1 teaspoon fresh rosemary, chopped
- Salt and pepper to taste
- 1 tablespoon balsamic vinegar (optional)
- 1 tablespoon fresh parsley, chopped (optional)

Instructions

1. Preheat the oven to 400 degrees Fahrenheit (200 degrees Celsius) and line a baking sheet with parchment paper.
2. Combine the beet wedges, olive oil, thyme, rosemary, salt, and pepper in a large mixing bowl.
3. Spread the beets out in a single layer on the prepared baking sheet.
4. Roast the beets in a preheated oven for 40-45 minutes, rotating halfway through, until soft and caramelized on the edges.
5. Remove from the oven and sprinkle with balsamic vinegar, if desired.
6. Garnish with fresh parsley and serve warm.

Nutrition Information (Per Serving):

Calories: 130 Protein: 2g Carbohydrates: 15g Fat: 7g Fiber: 4g Sodium: 160mg Sugar: 10g

Carrot and Apple Slaw

Prep Time: 10 minutes

Serving: 4

Ingredients

- 2 large carrots, grated
- 1 large apple, julienned or grated
- 1/4 cup of raisins or dried cranberries (optional)
- 2 tablespoons fresh lemon juice
- 2 tablespoons olive oil
- 1 teaspoon honey or maple syrup
- 1 tablespoon fresh parsley, chopped (optional)
- Salt and pepper to taste
- 1/4 cup of toasted sunflower seeds (optional for crunch)

Instructions

1. Add the grated carrots, apples, raisins, or dried cranberries in a large mixing bowl.
2. In a small mixing bowl, combine the lemon juice, olive oil, honey or maple syrup, salt, and pepper to make the dressing.
3. Toss the carrot and apple mixture with the dressing until well combined.
4. Garnish with fresh parsley and roasted sunflower seeds if preferred.
5. Serve immediately or chill for 15 minutes to let the flavors combine.

Nutrition Information (Per Serving):

Calories: 150 Protein: 2g Carbohydrates: 20g Fat: 7g Fiber: 4g Sodium: 70mg Sugar: 14g

Stuffed Bell Peppers with Quinoa

Prep Time: 15 minutes

Cook Time: 35-40 minutes

Serving: 4

Ingredients

- 4 large bell peppers (any color), tops cut off and seeds removed
- 1 cup of cooked quinoa
- 1/2 cup of black beans, rinsed and drained
- 1/2 cup of corn kernels (fresh or frozen)
- 1/2 cup of diced tomatoes
- 1/4 cup of red onion, finely chopped
- 2 tablespoons fresh cilantro, chopped
- 1 teaspoon ground cumin
- 1 teaspoon smoked paprika
- 1/4 teaspoon ground turmeric
- Salt and pepper to taste
- 1 tablespoon olive oil
- 1/4 cup of shredded cheese (optional for topping)

Instructions

1. Preheat the oven to 375°F (190° C). Lightly butter a baking dish and leave aside.
2. Combine the cooked quinoa, black beans, corn, diced tomatoes, red onion, cilantro, cumin, smoked paprika, turmeric, salt, and pepper in a large mixing bowl. Stir well to mix.
3. Drizzle olive oil into the bell peppers and season gently with salt.
4. Stuff each bell pepper with the quinoa mixture, carefully pushing it down to fill it.
5. Place the filled peppers upright in the prepared baking dish. Cover with foil and bake for 30-35 minutes, until the peppers are cooked.
6. If using cheese, remove the foil in the last 5 minutes of roasting and sprinkle it on top of each pepper. Bake uncovered until the cheese is melted and bubbling.
7. Remove from the oven and let it cool for a few minutes before serving.

Nutrition Information (Per Serving):

Calories: 220 Protein: 7g Carbohydrates: 34g Fat: 8g Fiber: 6g Sodium: 240mg Sugar: 6g

Roasted Eggplant with Tahini

Prep Time: 10 minutes

Cook Time: 25-30 minutes

Serving: 4

Ingredients

- 2 medium eggplants, sliced into 1/2-inch rounds
- 2 tablespoons olive oil
- 1/4 teaspoon ground cumin
- Salt and pepper to taste
- 1/4 cup of tahini
- 2 tablespoons fresh lemon juice
- 1 garlic clove, minced
- 2 tablespoons water (more if needed to thin the sauce)
- 1 tablespoon fresh parsley, chopped (optional)
- 1/4 teaspoon smoked paprika (optional for garnish)

Instructions

1. Preheat the oven to 400 degrees Fahrenheit (200 degrees Celsius) and line a baking sheet with parchment paper.
2. Place the eggplant slices on a baking pan and brush with olive oil on both sides. Season with cumin, salt, and pepper.
3. Roast the eggplant in a preheated oven for 25-30 minutes, turning halfway through, until golden brown and soft.
4. While the eggplant is roasting, mix the tahini, lemon juice, garlic, and water in a small bowl. Adjust the water to the desired consistency and season with salt to taste.
5. Place the slices on a serving plate and sprinkle with tahini sauce when the eggplant is done.
6. Garnish with fresh parsley and smoked paprika, if preferred.
7. Serve warm and enjoy!

Nutrition Information (Per Serving):

Calories: 180 Protein: 3g Carbohydrates: 12g Fat: 14g Fiber: 6g Sodium: 130mg Sugar: 3g

CHAPTER 3: SOUP AND SALAD

Sweet Potato and Ginger Soup

Prep Time: 10 minutes **Cook Time:** 25-30 minutes **Serving:** 4

Ingredients

- 2 large sweet potatoes, peeled and diced
- 1 medium onion, chopped
- 1 tablespoon fresh ginger, grated
- 2 garlic cloves, minced
- 1 tablespoon olive oil or coconut oil
- 4 cups of vegetable broth (or water)
- 1/2 teaspoon ground turmeric
- 1/4 teaspoon ground cumin (optional)
- Salt and pepper to taste
- 1/4 cup of coconut milk (optional for creaminess)
- Fresh cilantro or parsley for garnish (optional)

Instructions

1. In a large saucepan, warm the olive oil over medium heat. Sauté the chopped onion for 3-4 minutes, until softened.
2. Stir in the ginger and garlic and simmer for another minute until fragrant.
3. Combine the chopped sweet potatoes, turmeric, cumin (if using), salt, and pepper. Stir well to mix.
4. Add the veggie broth and bring to a boil. Reduce the heat and let the soup simmer for 20-25 minutes or until the sweet potatoes are cooked.
5. After softening the sweet potatoes, use an immersion blender to purée the soup until smooth. Alternatively, transfer the soup to a blender in batches and purée.
6. If preferred, stir in the coconut milk for an additional creamy texture.
7. Taste and adjust the seasoning as required. Garnish with fresh cilantro or parsley and serve warm.

Nutrition Information (Per Serving):

Calories: 190 Protein: 3g Carbohydrates: 35g Fat: 6g Fiber: 5g Sodium: 380mg Sugar: 9g

Hearty Lentil Stew

Prep Time: 10 minutes **Cook Time:** 40-45 minutes **Serving: 4**

Ingredients

- 1 cup of dried green or brown lentils, rinsed
- 1 medium onion, chopped
- 2 garlic cloves, minced
- 2 carrots, peeled and diced
- 2 celery stalks, diced
- 1 medium potato, diced (optional)
- 1 can (14.5 oz) diced tomatoes
- 4 cups of vegetable broth
- 1 tablespoon olive oil
- 1 teaspoon ground cumin
- 1/2 teaspoon ground turmeric
- 1/4 teaspoon smoked paprika
- Salt and pepper to taste
- 1 tablespoon fresh lemon juice (optional)
- Fresh parsley for garnish

Instructions

1. In a large saucepan, warm the olive oil over medium heat. Sauté the chopped onion, carrots, and celery for 5-6 minutes until the veggies soften.
2. Add the garlic, cumin, turmeric, and smoked paprika and simmer for another minute or until fragrant.
3. Combine the rinsed lentils, diced tomatoes, and vegetable broth. Stir well to mix.
4. Bring the mixture to a boil, lower to a low heat, and simmer uncovered for 30-35 minutes or until the lentils are cooked. If using, include the chopped potato halfway through the cooking time.
5. When the lentils are thoroughly cooked and the stew has thickened, season with salt, pepper, and a squeeze of fresh lemon juice for brightness (optional).
6. Ladle the stew into bowls, top with fresh parsley, and serve warm.

Nutrition Information (Per Serving):

Calories: 250 Protein: 12g Carbohydrates: 40g Fat: 5g Fiber: 15g Sodium: 500mg Sugar: 6g

Chicken and Vegetable Soup

Prep Time: 10 minutes

Cook Time: 30 minutes

Serving: 4

Ingredients

- 2 boneless, skinless chicken breasts (about 1 pound)
- 1 medium onion, chopped
- 2 garlic cloves, minced
- 2 carrots, peeled and sliced
- 2 celery stalks, sliced
- 1 zucchini, diced
- 1 cup of fresh spinach, chopped
- 6 cups of low-sodium chicken broth
- 1 tablespoon olive oil
- 1 teaspoon dried thyme
- 1/2 teaspoon dried oregano
- Salt and pepper to taste
- 1 tablespoon fresh lemon juice (optional)
- Fresh parsley, chopped (optional for garnish)

Instructions

1. In a large saucepan, warm the olive oil over medium heat. Sauté the chopped onion, carrots, and celery for 5-6 minutes, until softened.
2. Add the garlic and simmer for another minute or until fragrant.
3. Pour in the chicken broth and bring it to a boil.
4. Combine the chicken breasts, thyme, oregano, salt, and pepper. Reduce the heat to low, cover, and simmer for 15-20 minutes or until the chicken is well cooked.
5. Remove the chicken from the saucepan and shred it using two forks. Return the shredded chicken to the pot.
6. Add the zucchini and spinach to the broth and simmer for 5-7 minutes or until soft.
7. If preferred, add some fresh lemon juice for extra brightness.
8. Ladle the soup into bowls, top with fresh parsley, and serve warm.

Nutrition Information (Per Serving):

Calories: 250 Protein: 25g Carbohydrates: 12g Fat: 10g Fiber: 3g Sodium: 400mg Sugar: 4g

Tomato and White Bean Soup

Prep Time: 10 minutes

Cook Time: 25 minutes

Serving: 4

Ingredients

- 1 can (15 oz) white beans rinsed and drained
- 1 can (14.5 oz) diced tomatoes
- 1 small onion, chopped
- 2 garlic cloves, minced
- 1 tablespoon olive oil
- 4 cups of vegetable broth (or water)
- 1 teaspoon dried basil
- 1/2 teaspoon dried oregano
- 1/4 teaspoon red pepper flakes (optional)
- Salt and pepper to taste
- 1 tablespoon balsamic vinegar (optional)
- Fresh parsley or basil for garnish

Instructions

1. In a large saucepan, warm the olive oil over medium heat. Sauté the chopped onion for 4-5 minutes, until softened.
2. Add the garlic and simmer for another minute or until fragrant.
3. Add the chopped tomatoes, white beans, vegetable broth, dried basil, oregano, red pepper flakes (if desired), salt, and pepper.
4. Bring the soup to a boil, lower to low heat, and simmer for 15-20 minutes to let the flavors mingle.
5. If preferred, add the balsamic vinegar to enhance the taste.
6. Taste and adjust the seasoning as required. Ladle the soup into dishes and top with fresh parsley or basil.
7. Serve warm and enjoy!

Nutrition Information (Per Serving):

Calories: 180 Protein: 8g Carbohydrates: 26gFat: 4g Fiber: 7g Sodium: 450mg Sugar: 6g

Carrot and Coriander Soup

Prep Time: 10 minutes

Cook Time: 25 minutes

Serving: 4

Ingredients

- 1 tablespoon olive oil
- 1 onion, chopped
- 4 large carrots, peeled and chopped
- 2 garlic cloves, minced
- 1 teaspoon ground coriander
- 1/2 teaspoon ground cumin (optional)
- 4 cups of vegetable broth (or water)
- Salt and pepper to taste
- 1/4 cup of fresh cilantro (coriander) leaves, chopped
- 1 tablespoon fresh lemon juice (optional)

Instructions

1. In a large saucepan, warm the olive oil over medium heat. Sauté the chopped onion for 4-5 minutes, until softened.
2. Cook for another minute, stirring in the garlic, ground coriander, and cumin (if using), until fragrant.
3. Combine the diced carrots and vegetable broth. Bring the mixture to a boil, then lower it to a simmer for 20-25 minutes until the carrots are cooked.
4. Using an immersion blender, purée the soup until smooth. Alternatively, add the soup to a blender in batches and puree.
5. Mix in the fresh cilantro and lemon juice (if using). Taste and season with salt and pepper as required.
6. Serve warm, topped with additional fresh cilantro.

Nutrition Information (Per Serving):

Calories: 130 Protein: 2g Carbohydrates: 18g Fat: 5g Fiber: 5g Sodium: 380mg Sugar: 9g

Creamy Butternut Squash Soup

Prep Time: 10 minutes

Cook Time: 30 minutes

Serving: 4

Ingredients

- 1 medium butternut squash, peeled, seeded, and diced
- 1 medium onion, chopped
- 2 garlic cloves, minced
- 1 tablespoon olive oil or coconut oil
- 4 cups of vegetable broth
- 1/2 teaspoon ground cinnamon
- 1/4 teaspoon ground nutmeg
- Salt and pepper to taste
- 1/2 cup of coconut milk (optional for added creaminess)
- Fresh parsley or cilantro for garnish (optional)

Instructions

1. In a large saucepan, warm the olive oil over medium heat. Sauté the chopped onion for 4-5 minutes, until softened.
2. Add the garlic and simmer for another minute or until fragrant.
3. Combine the chopped butternut squash, vegetable broth, cinnamon, nutmeg, salt, and pepper.
4. Bring the mixture to a boil, lower to low heat, and cook for 20-25 minutes until the squash is soft.
5. Using an immersion blender, purée the soup until smooth. Alternatively, transfer the soup to a blender in stages and purée until smooth.
6. If preferred, stir in the coconut milk for an extra creamy texture.
7. Taste and adjust the seasoning as required. Garnish with fresh cilantro or parsley and serve warm.

Nutrition Information (Per Serving):

Calories: 180 Protein: 3g Carbohydrates: 28g Fat: 7g Fiber: 5g Sodium: 380mg Sugar: 8g

Pea and Mint Soup

Prep Time: 10 minutes

Cook Time: 15 minutes

Serving: 4

Ingredients

- 1 tablespoon olive oil
- 1 small onion, chopped
- 2 garlic cloves, minced
- 4 cups of frozen or fresh peas
- 4 cups of vegetable broth
- 1/4 cup of fresh mint leaves, chopped
- 1 tablespoon fresh lemon juice (optional)
- Salt and pepper to taste
- Fresh mint leaves for garnish (optional)

Instructions

1. In a large saucepan, warm the olive oil over medium heat. Sauté the chopped onion for 4-5 minutes, until softened.
2. Stir in the garlic and simmer for another minute until fragrant.
3. Bring the peas and vegetable broth to a boil. Reduce the heat and let the peas simmer for 10 minutes, until soft.
4. Remove from the fire and add the chopped mint and lemon juice (if using).
5. Using an immersion blender, purée the soup until smooth. Alternatively, transfer the soup to a blender in stages and purée until smooth.
6. Taste and season with salt and pepper as required.
7. Serve warm, topped with fresh mint leaves if preferred.

Nutrition Information (Per Serving)

Calories: 170 Protein: 7g Carbohydrates: 28g Fat: 5g Fiber: 8g Sodium: 380mg Sugar: 10g

Spicy Black Bean Soup

Prep Time: 10 minutes

Cook Time: 25 minutes

Serving: 4

Ingredients

- 1 tablespoon olive oil
- 1 small onion, chopped
- 3 garlic cloves, minced
- 1 jalapeño, seeded and chopped (optional for spice)
- 2 cans (15 oz each) black beans, rinsed and drained
- 1 can (14.5 oz) diced tomatoes
- 4 cups of vegetable broth (or water)
- 1 teaspoon ground cumin
- 1/2 teaspoon smoked paprika
- 1/4 teaspoon chili powder (optional for extra heat)
- Salt and pepper to taste
- Juice of 1 lime
- Fresh cilantro for garnish (optional)

Instructions

1. In a large saucepan, warm the olive oil over medium heat. Sauté the chopped onion for 4-5 minutes, until softened.
2. Cook the garlic and jalapeño for another minute until fragrant.
3. Add the black beans, chopped tomatoes, vegetable broth, cumin, smoked paprika, chili powder (if desired), salt, and pepper.
4. Bring the mixture to a boil, lower to low heat, and cook for 15-20 minutes to let the flavors mingle.
5. Use an immersion blender to partly puree the soup while retaining some texture, or transfer half of the soup to a blender, puree, and then stir back into the saucepan.
6. Stir in the lime juice and season to taste.
7. Serve warm, topped with fresh cilantro if preferred.

Nutrition Information (Per Serving):

Calories: 220 Protein: 10g Carbohydrates: 37g Fat: 4g Fiber: 12g Sodium: 500mg Sugar: 5g

Broccoli and Almond Soup

Prep Time: 10 minutes

Cook Time: 20 minutes

Serving: 4

Ingredients

- 1 tablespoon olive oil
- 1 small onion, chopped
- 2 garlic cloves, minced
- 4 cups of broccoli florets (about 1 large head of broccoli)
- 1/4 cup of blanched almonds
- 4 cups of vegetable broth
- 1/2 teaspoon ground cumin
- Salt and pepper to taste
- 1/4 cup of unsweetened almond milk (optional for creaminess)
- 1 tablespoon fresh lemon juice (optional)
- Slivered almonds for garnish (optional)

Instructions

1. In a large saucepan, warm the olive oil over medium heat. Sauté the chopped onion for 4-5 minutes, until softened.
2. Add the garlic and simmer for another minute or until fragrant.
3. Stir in the broccoli florets and blanched almonds, then simmer for 2-3 minutes, stirring periodically.
4. Pour in the veggie broth and bring to a boil. Reduce the heat to a simmer for 15 minutes or until the broccoli is soft.
5. Puree the soup with an immersion blender until smooth or in batches in a blender until creamy.
6. Add almond milk for creaminess, and season with salt, pepper, and lemon juice if preferred.
7. Ladle the soup into bowls and top with slivered almonds, if preferred. Serve warm.

Nutrition Information (Per Serving):

Calories: 180 Protein: 6g Carbohydrates: 16g Fat: 10g Fiber: 6g Sodium: 350mg Sugar: 4g

Mushroom and Thyme Stew

Prep Time: 10 minutes

Cook Time: 30 minutes

Serving: 4

Ingredients

- 2 tablespoons olive oil
- 1 medium onion, chopped
- 3 garlic cloves, minced
- 16 oz (450 g) mushrooms, sliced
- 2 carrots, peeled and sliced
- 2 celery stalks, chopped
- 4 cups of vegetable broth
- 1 tablespoon fresh thyme leaves (or 1 teaspoon dried thyme)
- 1/2 teaspoon smoked paprika
- 1 tablespoon soy sauce or tamari (for gluten-free)
- Salt and pepper to taste
- 1 tablespoon fresh parsley, chopped (optional for garnish)

Instructions

1. In a large saucepan, warm the olive oil over medium heat. Sauté the chopped onion for 4-5 minutes, until softened.
2. Add the garlic and simmer for another minute or until fragrant.
3. Mix in the mushrooms, carrots, and celery. Cook for 6-8 minutes, stirring periodically, until the veggies soften and the mushrooms release moisture.
4. Combine the vegetable broth, thyme, smoked paprika, soy sauce, salt, and pepper. Bring the mixture to a boil, then lower to a simmer for 20 minutes to let the flavors combine and the veggies soften.
5. Taste and adjust the seasoning as required. Ladle the stew into dishes and top with fresh parsley, if preferred.
6. Serve warm and enjoy!

Nutrition Information (Per Serving):

Calories: 180 Protein: 6g Carbohydrates: 20g Fat: 8g Fiber: 4g Sodium: 450mg Sugar: 6g

Mediterranean Chickpea Salad

Prep Time: 10 minutes

Serving: 4

Ingredients

- 1 can (15 oz) chickpeas, rinsed and drained
- 1 cup of cucumber, diced
- 1 cup of cherry tomatoes, halved
- 1/4 cup of red onion, finely chopped
- 1/4 cup of Kalamata olives, pitted and sliced
- 1/4 cup of feta cheese, crumbled (optional for vegan)
- 2 tablespoons fresh parsley, chopped
- 2 tablespoons fresh lemon juice
- 2 tablespoons olive oil
- 1 teaspoon dried oregano
- Salt and pepper to taste

Instructions

1. Add chickpeas, cucumber, cherry tomatoes, red onion, olives, feta cheese (if using), and parsley in a large mixing bowl.
2. To make the dressing, combine lemon juice, olive oil, oregano, salt, and pepper in a small mixing dish.
3. Toss the chickpea mixture with the dressing until well combined.
4. Serve immediately or chill for 15-30 minutes to let the flavors combine.
5. If preferred, garnish with more parsley or feta.

Nutrition Information (Per Serving):

Calories: 220 Protein: 7g Carbohydrates: 20g Fat: 12g Fiber: 6g Sodium: 320mg Sugar: 4g

Cucumber and Dill Salad

Prep Time: 10 minutes

Serving: 4

Ingredients

- 2 large cucumbers, thinly sliced
- 1/4 cup of red onion, thinly sliced
- 2 tablespoons fresh dill, chopped
- 2 tablespoons apple cider vinegar
- 1 tablespoon olive oil
- 1 teaspoon honey or maple syrup (optional)
- Salt and pepper to taste
- 1 tablespoon fresh lemon juice (optional)

Instructions

1. Add thinly sliced cucumbers, red onion, and fresh dill in a large mixing bowl.
2. In a small mixing bowl, combine the apple cider vinegar, olive oil, honey (if using), salt, pepper, and lemon juice (if using).
3. Toss the cucumber mixture with the dressing until well-coated.
4. Enable the salad to rest for 10-15 minutes to enable the flavors to mingle before serving immediately.
5. If desired, garnish with more fresh dill.

Nutrition Information (Per Serving):

Calories: 60 Protein: 1g Carbohydrates: 7g Fat: 3g Fiber: 1g Sodium: 50mg Sugar: 3g

Quinoa and Roasted Beet Salad

Prep Time: 10 minutes

Cook Time: 40 minutes

Serving: 4

Ingredients

- 1 cup of quinoa, rinsed
- 2 medium beets, peeled and diced
- 2 tablespoons olive oil, divided
- 1/4 cup of feta cheese, crumbled (optional for vegan)
- 1/4 cup of walnuts, toasted and chopped
- 1/4 cup of fresh parsley, chopped
- 2 tablespoons fresh lemon juice
- 1 teaspoon Dijon mustard
- Salt and pepper to taste
- 1 tablespoon balsamic vinegar (optional)

Instructions

1. Preheat the oven to 400 °F (200 °C). Toss chopped beets with 1 tablespoon olive oil, salt, and pepper. Place the beets on a baking sheet and roast for 35-40 minutes or until cooked, stirring halfway through.
2. While the beets roast, prepare the quinoa. In a medium saucepan, mix the quinoa and 2 cups of water. Bring to a boil, then decrease the heat, cover, and cook for 15 minutes or until the quinoa is soft and the water has been absorbed. Fluff the quinoa with a fork, then put aside to chill.
3. In a small mixing bowl, combine the remaining 1 tablespoon olive oil, lemon juice, Dijon mustard, and balsamic vinegar (if using).
4. Add cooked quinoa, roasted beets, feta cheese (if using), toasted walnuts, and fresh parsley in a large mixing bowl.
5. Toss the salad with the dressing until well combined. Season with salt and pepper to taste.
6. Serve immediately or chill for 15-30 minutes to let the flavors combine.

Nutrition Information (Per Serving):

Calories: 270 Protein: 7g Carbohydrates: 28g Fat: 15g Fiber: 5g Sodium: 180mg Sugar: 6g

Tomato and Turmeric Stew

Prep Time: 10 minutes

Cook Time: 25-30 minutes

Serving: 4

Ingredients

- 2 tablespoons olive oil
- 1 medium onion, chopped
- 3 garlic cloves, minced
- 1 tablespoon fresh ginger, grated
- 1 teaspoon ground turmeric
- 1/2 teaspoon ground cumin
- 1/2 teaspoon smoked paprika (optional)
- 4 large tomatoes, chopped (or 1 can of diced tomatoes)
- 1 can (15 oz) chickpeas, drained and rinsed
- 4 cups of vegetable broth
- 1 cup of spinach, chopped
- Salt and pepper to taste
- 1 tablespoon fresh lemon juice (optional)
- Fresh cilantro or parsley for garnish

Instructions:

1. In a large saucepan, warm the olive oil over medium heat. Sauté the chopped onion for 4-5 minutes, until softened.
2. Stir in the garlic, ginger, turmeric, cumin, and smoked paprika (if using) and simmer for another minute until aromatic.
3. Cook the chopped tomatoes for 5-7 minutes, stirring periodically, until they break down and release juice.
4. Stir in the chickpeas and veggie broth. Bring the stew to a boil, then lower to a simmer for 15-20 minutes to let the flavors combine.
5. Add the chopped spinach and simmer for 2-3 minutes or until wilted.
6. Season with salt, pepper, and fresh lemon juice, if preferred.
7. Ladle the stew into dishes and top with fresh cilantro or parsley. Serve warm.

Nutrition Information (Per Serving):

Calories: 220 Protein: 8g Carbohydrates: 28g Fat: 8g Fiber: 8g Sodium: 400mg Sugar: 8g

Lentil and Spinach Soup

Prep Time: 10 minutes

Cook Time: 30 minutes

Serving: 4

Ingredients:

- 1 tablespoon olive oil
- 1 small onion, chopped
- 2 garlic cloves, minced
- 1 carrot, diced
- 1 celery stalk, diced
- 1 cup of dried green or brown lentils, rinsed
- 4 cups of vegetable broth
- 1 can (14.5 oz) diced tomatoes
- 1 teaspoon ground cumin
- 1/2 teaspoon ground turmeric
- Salt and pepper to taste
- 2 cups of fresh spinach, chopped
- 1 tablespoon fresh lemon juice (optional)
- Fresh parsley for garnish (optional)

Instructions:

1. In a large saucepan, warm the olive oil over medium heat. Sauté the onion, carrot, and celery for 4-5 minutes, until softened.
2. Cook for another minute until the garlic, cumin, and turmeric are aromatic.
3. Combine the lentils, vegetable broth, and diced tomatoes. Bring to a boil, then decrease heat and cook for 25-30 minutes or until the lentils are cooked.
4. Stir in the chopped spinach and simmer for 2-3 minutes or until wilted.
5. Season to taste with salt, pepper, and a dash of fresh lemon juice.
6. Ladle the soup into bowls, top with fresh parsley, and serve warm.

Nutrition Information (Per Serving):

Calories: 240 Protein: 12g Carbohydrates: 34g Fat: 6g Fiber: 13g Sodium: 450mg Sugar: 6g

Roasted Beet and Goat Cheese Salad

Prep Time: 10 minutes

Cook Time: 40 minutes (for roasting beets)

Serving: 4

Ingredients:

- 4 medium beets, peeled and diced
- 2 tablespoons olive oil, divided
- Salt and pepper to taste
- 4 cups of mixed greens (such as arugula or spinach)
- 1/4 cup of crumbled goat cheese
- 1/4 cup of walnuts, toasted and chopped
- 1 tablespoon balsamic vinegar
- 1 teaspoon Dijon mustard
- 1 teaspoon honey or maple syrup (optional)

Instructions:

1. Preheat the oven to 400 °F (200 °C). Toss chopped beets with 1 tablespoon olive oil, salt, and pepper. Spread them evenly over a baking sheet.
2. Roast the beets for 35-40 minutes, until tender, stirring halfway through. Once done, remove it from the oven and let it cool slightly.
3. While the beets roast, make the dressing by whisking together the remaining tablespoon of olive oil, balsamic vinegar, Dijon mustard, and honey (if using) in a small bowl.
4. Toss the mixed greens in a large bowl with the dressing until completely coated.
5. Divide the dressed greens among plates, then top with roasted beets, crumbled goat cheese, and toasted walnuts.
6. Serve immediately and enjoy!

Nutrition Information (Per Serving):

Calories: 220 Protein: 6g Carbohydrates: 16g Fat: 16g Fiber: 4g Sodium: 180mg Sugar: 7g

Chicken Noodle Soup with Turmeric

Prep Time: 10 minutes

Cook Time: 25 minutes

Serving: 4

Ingredients

- 1 tablespoon olive oil
- 1 small onion, chopped
- 2 garlic cloves, minced
- 2 medium carrots, sliced
- 2 celery stalks, sliced
- 1 teaspoon ground turmeric
- 1/2 teaspoon ground ginger (optional)
- 6 cups of low-sodium chicken broth
- 2 boneless, skinless chicken breasts
- 1 cup of whole wheat or gluten-free noodles
- 1/2 teaspoon dried thyme
- Salt and pepper to taste
- 2 tablespoons fresh parsley, chopped (optional)
- Fresh lemon wedges (optional for serving)

Instructions

1. In a large saucepan, warm the olive oil over medium heat. Sauté the onion, carrots, and celery for 4-5 minutes, until softened.
2. Add the garlic, turmeric, and ground ginger (if using) and simmer for another minute or until aromatic.
3. Add the chicken broth and bring to a boil. Add the chicken breasts, decrease the heat, and cook for 15 minutes or until well done.
4. Remove the chicken from the pot, shred it with two forks, and add it to the soup.
5. Stir in the noodles and dried thyme. Simmer for 6-8 minutes or until the noodles are soft.
6. Season with salt and pepper to taste. To enhance flavor, stir in fresh parsley.
7. Serve the soup warm, with a squeeze of fresh lemon juice if preferred.

Nutrition Information (Per Serving):

Calories: 280 Protein: 25g Carbohydrates: 30g Fat: 7g Fiber: 4g Sodium: 450mg Sugar: 4g

Vegetable Minestrone

Prep Time: 10 minutes **Cook Time:** 30 minutes **Serving: 4**

Ingredients

- 1 tablespoon olive oil
- 1 small onion, chopped
- 2 garlic cloves, minced
- 2 medium carrots, diced
- 2 celery stalks, diced
- 1 zucchini, diced
- 1 cup of green beans, trimmed and cut into 1-inch pieces
- 1 can (14.5 oz) diced tomatoes
- 4 cups of vegetable broth
- 1 can (15 oz) cannellini beans, rinsed and drained
- 1/2 cup of small pasta (whole wheat or gluten-free)
- 1 teaspoon dried basil
- 1/2 teaspoon dried oregano
- Salt and pepper to taste
- 2 cups of fresh spinach or kale, chopped
- Fresh parsley or basil for garnish (optional)

Instructions

1. In a large saucepan, warm the olive oil over medium heat. Sauté the onion, carrots, and celery for 4-5 minutes, until softened.
2. Add the garlic and simmer for another minute or until fragrant.
3. Combine the chopped zucchini, green beans, diced tomatoes, vegetable broth, cannellini beans, dry basil, and oregano. Bring to a boil, decrease heat, and let simmer for 15 minutes.
4. Add the pasta to the saucepan and simmer for 8-10 minutes or until cooked.
5. Add the chopped spinach or kale and simmer for 2-3 minutes or until wilted. Season with salt and pepper to taste.
6. Ladle the soup into bowls and serve with fresh parsley or basil, if preferred. Serve warm.

Nutrition Information (Per Serving):

Calories: 250 Protein: 10g Carbohydrates: 40g Fat: 5g Fiber: 9g Sodium: 380mg Sugar: 7g

CHAPTER 4: FISH AND SEAFOOD

Baked Salmon with Dill and Lemon

Prep Time: 5 minutes **Cook Time:** 15-20 minutes **Serving:** 4

Ingredients

- 4 salmon fillets
- 2 tablespoons olive oil
- 2 tablespoons fresh dill, chopped
- 1 lemon, thinly sliced
- 1 tablespoon fresh lemon juice
- 2 garlic cloves, minced
- Salt and pepper to taste

Instructions

1. Preheat the oven to 375°F (190° C). Cover a baking sheet with parchment paper or gently oil it.
2. Place the salmon fillets on the prepared baking sheet.
3. Mix the olive oil, garlic, fresh dill, and lemon juice in a small bowl. Season with salt and pepper to taste.
4. Brush the salmon fillets with olive oil, ensuring they are well covered.
5. Place lemon wedges on top of each salmon fillet.
6. Bake in the oven for 15-20 minutes until the salmon is fully cooked and readily flaked with a fork.
7. Remove from the oven and serve immediately, topped with more fresh dill and lemon wedges if preferred.

Nutrition Information (Per Serving):

Calories: 320 Protein: 34g Carbohydrates: 2g Fat: 19g Fiber: 0g Sodium: 150mg Sugar: 0g

Grilled Tuna with Avocado Salsa

Prep Time: 10 minutes

Cook Time: 6-8 minutes

Serving: 4

Ingredients:

- For the Grilled Tuna:
- 4 tuna steaks (about 6 oz each)
- 2 tablespoons olive oil
- 1 tablespoon fresh lemon juice
- 1 garlic clove, minced
- Salt and pepper to taste
- For the Avocado Salsa:
- 1 ripe avocado, diced
- 1/2 cup of cherry tomatoes, halved
- 1/4 cup of red onion, finely chopped
- 1 tablespoon fresh cilantro, chopped
- 1 tablespoon fresh lime juice
- Salt and pepper to taste

Instructions

1. Combine the olive oil, lemon juice, garlic, salt, and pepper in a small bowl.
2. Brush the marinade over the tuna steaks, covering both sides. Allow them to sit for 5 minutes while you prepare the grill.
3. Preheat the grill or grill pan to medium-high heat.
4. Grill the tuna steaks for 3-4 minutes on each side, depending on their thickness and desired amount of doneness. For medium-rare, the center should remain pink. Remove off the grill and put aside.
5. Add chopped avocado, cherry tomatoes, red onion, cilantro, lime juice, salt, and pepper in a medium mixing bowl. Toss lightly to combine.
6. Plate the grilled tuna steaks and top with avocado salsa. Serve immediately.

Nutrition Information (Per Serving):

Calories: 320 Protein: 34g Carbohydrates: 8g Fat: 18g Fiber: 4g Sodium: 180mg Sugar: 1g

Garlic Shrimp with Zucchini Noodles

Prep Time: 10 minutes

Cook Time: 10 minutes

Serving: 4

Ingredients

- 1 pound large shrimp, peeled and deveined
- 3 medium zucchinis, spiralized into noodles
- 3 garlic cloves, minced
- 2 tablespoons olive oil
- 1 tablespoon fresh lemon juice
- 1/4 teaspoon red pepper flakes (optional)
- Salt and pepper to taste
- Fresh parsley, chopped (optional for garnish)
- Lemon wedges for serving (optional)

Instructions

1. Spiralize the zucchini and leave aside. To make the noodles, use either a spiralizer or a vegetable peeler.
2. Heat 1 tablespoon olive oil in a large pan over medium heat. Sauté the garlic and red pepper flakes (if using) for 1 minute or until aromatic.
3. Season the shrimp in the pan with salt and pepper. Cook for 2-3 minutes on each side or until the shrimp is pink and cooked. Remove the shrimp from the skillet and put it aside.
4. Combine the remaining tablespoon of olive oil in the same pan with the zucchini noodles. Sauté the noodles for 2-3 minutes until soft but somewhat crunchy.
5. Stir in the fresh lemon juice and season with salt and pepper as required.
6. Return the cooked shrimp to the pan and stir in the zucchini noodles. Garnish with fresh parsley and serve immediately with lemon wedges on the side.

Nutrition Information (Per Serving):

Calories: 210 Protein: 25g Carbohydrates: 7g Fat: 10g Fiber: 2g Sodium: 300mg Sugar: 4g

Broiled Cod with Turmeric and Garlic

Prep Time: 10 minutes

Cook Time: 8-10 minutes

Serving: 4

Ingredients

- 4 cod fillets (about 6 oz each)
- 2 tablespoons olive oil
- 1 teaspoon ground turmeric
- 3 garlic cloves, minced
- 1 tablespoon fresh lemon juice
- Salt and pepper to taste
- Fresh parsley, chopped (optional for garnish)
- Lemon wedges for serving (optional)

Instructions

1. Preheat your oven's broiler, prepare a baking sheet with parchment paper, or gently grease it.
2. Combine the olive oil, turmeric, garlic, lemon juice, salt, and pepper in a small mixing bowl.
3. Place the cod fillets on the prepared baking sheet and liberally apply the marinade on both sides.
4. Place the baking sheet in the broiler for 8-10 minutes or until the cod is well cooked and readily flaked with a fork. The time will vary according to the thickness of the fillets.
5. Remove the fish from the oven and serve with fresh parsley. Serve with lemon wedges on the side for an added kick of flavor.

Nutrition Information (Per Serving):

Calories: 220 Protein: 30g Carbohydrates: 2g Fat: 10g Fiber: 1g Sodium: 180mg Sugar: 0g

Seared Scallops with Cauliflower Purée

Prep Time: 10 minutes

Cook Time: 15 minutes

Serving: 4

Ingredients

- 12 large sea scallops
- 1 tablespoon olive oil
- Salt and pepper to taste
- 1 tablespoon fresh lemon juice (optional)
- Fresh parsley, chopped (optional for garnish)
- For the Cauliflower Purée:
- 1 medium head cauliflower, chopped into florets
- 2 tablespoons olive oil or butter
- 1/2 cup of unsweetened almond milk
- 2 garlic cloves, minced
- Salt and pepper to taste

Instructions

1. Steam the cauliflower florets for 10 to 12 minutes or until very soft. Once cooked, place in a blender or food processor.
2. Combine the olive oil or butter, almond milk, garlic, salt, and pepper in the blender. Blend until smooth and creamy. Set aside to stay warm.
3. Pat the scallops dry with paper towels before seasoning with salt and pepper.
4. Heat the olive oil in a large pan over medium-high heat. When the oil is heated, arrange the scallops in a single layer, taking care not to overcrowd the pan. Sear the scallops on each side for 2-3 minutes until golden brown.
5. Remove the scallops from the pan and sprinkle with lemon juice, if preferred.
6. To serve, ladle cauliflower purée onto plates and top with grilled scallops. Garnish with fresh parsley and serve immediately.

Nutrition Information (Per Serving):

Calories: 250 Carbohydrates: 12g Fiber: 4g Sugar: 3g

Turmeric Spiced Baked Tilapia

Prep Time: 10 minutes

Cook Time: 15 minutes

Serving: 4

Ingredients

- 4 tilapia fillets (about 6 oz each)
- 2 tablespoons olive oil
- 1 teaspoon ground turmeric
- 1/2 teaspoon ground cumin
- 1/2 teaspoon paprika
- 2 garlic cloves, minced
- 1 tablespoon fresh lemon juice
- Salt and pepper to taste
- Fresh cilantro or parsley, chopped (optional for garnish)
- Lemon wedges for serving (optional)

Instructions

1. Preheat the oven to 400°F (200°C). Line a baking sheet with parchment paper or gently oil it.
2. Mix the olive oil, turmeric, cumin, paprika, chopped garlic, lemon juice, salt, and pepper in a small bowl to make a marinade.
3. Rub the marinade onto the tilapia fillets, ensuring they are uniformly covered on both sides.
4. Place the fillets on the prepared baking sheet and bake for 12-15 minutes or until opaque and readily flaked with a fork.
5. Remove from the oven and serve with fresh cilantro or parsley. Serve lemon slices on the side for extra flavor.

Nutrition Information (Per Serving):

Calories: 220 Protein: 28g Carbohydrates: 2g Fat: 11g Fiber: 1g Sodium: 150mg Sugar: 0g

Lemon Herb Grilled Mackerel

Prep Time: 10 minutes

Cook Time: 10 minutes

Serving: 4

Ingredients

- 4 mackerel fillets (about 6 oz each)
- 2 tablespoons olive oil
- 2 tablespoons fresh lemon juice
- 2 garlic cloves, minced
- 1 tablespoon fresh parsley, chopped
- 1 tablespoon fresh thyme leaves (or 1/2 teaspoon dried thyme)
- Salt and pepper to taste
- Lemon wedges for serving

Instructions

1. Preheat the grill or grill pan to medium-high heat.
2. The marinade is made by whisking together olive oil, lemon juice, garlic, parsley, thyme, salt, and pepper in a small bowl.
3. Rub the marinade into the mackerel fillets, ensuring they are uniformly covered on both sides.
4. Place the fillets on the grill, skin side down, and cook for 4-5 minutes on each side until the fish is cooked through and easily flaked with a fork.
5. Remove from the grill and serve with lemon wedges for added taste.

Nutrition Information (Per Serving):

Calories: 280 Protein: 24g Carbohydrates: 2g Fat: 20g Fiber: 0g Sodium: 180mg Sugar: 0g

Smoked Salmon and Avocado Salad

Prep Time: 10 minutes

Serving: 4

Ingredients

- 4 cups of mixed greens (arugula, spinach, or lettuce)
- 8 oz smoked salmon, sliced
- 1 ripe avocado, diced
- 1/2 red onion, thinly sliced
- 1/4 cup of cucumber, diced
- 1 tablespoon capers (optional)
- 2 tablespoons olive oil
- 1 tablespoon fresh lemon juice
- Salt and pepper to taste
- Fresh dill for garnish (optional)

Instructions

1. In a large mixing bowl, combine the greens, red onion, cucumber, and capers (if using).
2. Place the smoked salmon and chopped avocado on top of the greens.
3. Combine the olive oil, lemon juice, salt, and pepper in a small bowl.
4. Drizzle the dressing over the salad and gently toss to mix.
5. Garnish with fresh dill if preferred and serve immediately.

Nutrition Information (Per Serving):

Calories: 250 Protein: 15g Carbohydrates: 8g Fat: 18g Fiber: 6g Sodium: 600mg Sugar: 1g

Pesto-Crusted Halibut

Prep Time: 10 minutes

Cook Time: 12-15 minutes

Serving: 4

Ingredients:

- 4 halibut fillets (about 6 oz each)
- 1/2 cup of fresh basil pesto
- 1/4 cup of almond flour
- 1 tablespoon olive oil
- Salt and pepper to taste
- Lemon wedges for serving (optional)

Instructions

1. Preheat the oven to 400 degrees Fahrenheit (200 degrees Celsius) and line a baking sheet with parchment paper.
2. Season the halibut fillets with salt and pepper on both sides.
3. Combine the basil pesto and almond flour in a small bowl to form a thick paste.
4. Spread the pesto mixture equally on top of each halibut fillet, gently pushing it down to adhere.
5. Drizzle olive oil over the fish fillets and lay them on the baking sheet.
6. Bake for 12-15 minutes or until the halibut is well cooked and readily flaked with a fork.
7. Serve with lemon wedges for an added blast of flavor.

Nutrition Information (Per Serving):

Calories: 320 Protein: 32g Carbohydrates: 4g Fat: 20g Fiber: 1g Sodium: 350mg Sugar: 0g

Coconut Curry Salmon

Prep Time: 10 minutes

Cook Time: 15 minutes

Serving: 4

Ingredients

- 4 salmon fillets (about 6 oz each)
- 1 tablespoon olive oil
- 1 small onion, chopped
- 2 garlic cloves, minced
- 1 tablespoon fresh ginger, grated
- 1 tablespoon red curry paste
- 1 can (14 oz) coconut milk (full-fat or light)
- 1 tablespoon fresh lime juice
- 1 tablespoon fresh cilantro, chopped (optional for garnish)
- Salt and pepper to taste
- Lime wedges for serving

Instructions

1. Heat the olive oil in a large pan over medium heat. Sauté the chopped onion for 3-4 minutes, until softened.
2. Add the garlic and ginger and simmer for another minute or until fragrant.
3. Add the red curry paste to the pan and whisk for 1 minute to combine the flavors.
4. Pour in the coconut milk, swirl to incorporate, and simmer.
5. Season the salmon fillets with salt and pepper and set them on the pan, skin side down. Spoon some of the coconut curry sauce onto the fillets.
6. Cover the pan and simmer for 10-12 minutes until the salmon is cooked and easily flaked with a fork.
7. Remove from the fire and mix in the fresh lime juice.
8. Serve the salmon with the coconut curry sauce, topped with fresh cilantro and lime wedges if preferred.

Nutrition Information (Per Serving): Fat: 12g Fiber: 1g Sodium: 180mg Sugar: 0g

Fish Tacos with Mango Salsa

Prep Time: 15 minutes **Cook Time:** 10 minutes **Serving: 4**

Ingredients:

- For the Fish:
- 4 white fish fillets
- 2 tablespoons olive oil
- 1 teaspoon ground cumin
- 1/2 teaspoon paprika
- 1/2 teaspoon ground turmeric
- Salt and pepper to taste
- 8 small corn or flour tortillas
- For the Mango Salsa:
- 1 ripe mango, diced
- 1/4 red onion, finely chopped
- 1 jalapeño, seeded and finely chopped
- 2 tablespoons fresh cilantro, chopped
- 1 tablespoon fresh lime juice
- Salt to taste

Instructions:

1. Mix diced mango, red onion, jalapeño, cilantro, lime juice, and salt in a medium bowl. Toss to blend, then put aside.
2. Pat the fish fillets dry and season with cumin, paprika, turmeric, salt, and pepper on both sides.
3. Heat the olive oil in a large pan over medium heat. Cook the fish for 3-4 minutes on each side or until it is opaque and readily flaked with a fork.
4. Once cooked, break the fish into bite-sized pieces.
5. Heat the tortillas in a dry skillet or microwave.
6. Divide the fish equally among the tortillas, then top with mango salsa.
7. If preferred, serve the tacos with extra lime wedges and fresh cilantro.

Nutrition Information (Per Serving - 2 tacos):

Calories: 320 Protein: 28g Carbohydrates: 26g Fat: 12g Fiber: 4g Sodium: 250mg Sugar: 7g

Pan-Seared Trout with Almonds

Prep Time: 10 minutes

Cook Time: 10 minutes

Serving: 4

Ingredients

- 4 trout fillets (about 6 oz each)
- 1/4 cup of sliced almonds, toasted
- 2 tablespoons olive oil
- 2 tablespoons fresh lemon juice
- 2 garlic cloves, minced
- 1 tablespoon fresh parsley, chopped
- Salt and pepper to taste
- Lemon wedges for serving (optional)

Instructions

1. Season the fish fillets with salt and pepper on both sides.
2. Heat the olive oil in a large pan over medium-high heat. Cook the trout fillets, skin side down, for 3-4 minutes until the skin is crispy.
3. Carefully rotate the fillets and cook for 2-3 minutes or until the fish flakes easily with a fork. Remove from the skillet and put aside.
4. In the same skillet, sauté the minced garlic for 1 minute, until fragrant.
5. Cook for another minute, stirring in the fresh lemon juice and roasted almonds until well warmed.
6. Remove from the heat and spread the almond mixture over the fish fillets.
7. Garnish with fresh parsley and serve with lemon wedges for an added punch of flavor.

Nutrition Information (Per Serving):

Calories: 290 Protein: 32g Carbohydrates: 3g Fat: 18g Fiber: 2g Sugar: 0g

Shrimp and Broccoli Stir-Fry

Prep Time: 10 minutes

Cook Time: 10 minutes

Serving: 4

Ingredients

- 1 pound large shrimp, peeled and deveined
- 3 cups of broccoli florets
- 2 tablespoons olive oil
- 3 garlic cloves, minced
- 1 tablespoon fresh ginger, grated
- 2 tablespoons low-sodium soy sauce
- 1 tablespoon rice vinegar
- 1 tablespoon honey or maple syrup
- 1 teaspoon sesame oil (optional for flavor)
- 1/4 teaspoon red pepper flakes (optional for heat)
- 2 green onions, chopped (optional for garnish)
- Sesame seeds for garnish (optional)

Instructions

1. Heat 1 tablespoon olive oil in a large pan or wok over medium-high heat. Cook the shrimp on each side for 2-3 minutes until pink and thoroughly done. Remove the shrimp from the skillet and put it aside.
2. In the same skillet, warm the remaining olive oil. Sauté the garlic and ginger for 1 minute, until fragrant.
3. Stir-fry the broccoli florets for 4-5 minutes, until tender yet crisp.
4. In a small mixing bowl, combine the soy sauce, rice vinegar, honey, sesame oil, and red pepper flakes (if using). Pour the sauce over the broccoli, stirring to coat.
5. Return the shrimp to the pan and stir everything together, cooking for another 1-2 minutes until well cooked.
6. If preferred, serve the stir-fry immediately, topped with chopped green onions and sesame seeds.

Nutrition Information (Per Serving):

Calories: 230 Protein: 26g Carbohydrates: 10g Fat: 10g Fiber: 3g Sodium: 480mg Sugar: 5g

CHAPTER 5: VEGAN AND VEGETARIAN

Vegan Lentil and Spinach Curry

Prep Time: 10 minutes **Cook Time:** 25-30 minutes **Serving:** 4

Ingredients

- 1 cup of dried lentils (green or brown), rinsed
- 1 tablespoon olive oil or coconut oil
- 1 onion, chopped
- 3 garlic cloves, minced
- 1 tablespoon fresh ginger, grated
- 1 tablespoon curry powder
- 1/2 teaspoon ground turmeric
- 1/2 teaspoon ground cumin
- 1 can (14.5 oz) diced tomatoes
- 4 cups of vegetable broth
- 2 cups of fresh spinach, chopped
- 1/4 cup of coconut milk (optional for creaminess)
- Salt and pepper to taste
- Fresh cilantro for garnish (optional)

Instructions

1. Warm the olive or coconut oil over medium heat in a large saucepan. Sauté the chopped onion for 4-5 minutes, until softened.
2. Cook for a further minute or until the garlic and ginger are aromatic.
3. Cook for 30 seconds to toast the curry powder, turmeric, and cumin.
4. Combine the lentils, diced tomatoes, and vegetable broth. Bring the mixture to a boil, then decrease the heat and cook for 20-25 minutes or until the lentils are cooked.
5. Stir in the fresh spinach and simmer for 2-3 minutes or until wilted.
6. Add coconut milk for extra creaminess and season with salt and pepper.
7. Serve the curry warm, topped with fresh cilantro if preferred.

Nutrition Information (Per Serving):

Calories: 280 Protein: 15g Carbohydrates: 40g Fat: 7g Fiber: 14g Sodium: 450mg Sugar: 6g

Vegan Stuffed Peppers with Quinoa

Prep Time: 15 minutes **Cook Time:** 35-40 minutes **Serving: 4**

Ingredients

- 4 large bell peppers (any color), tops cut off and seeds removed
- 1 cup of cooked quinoa
- 1 can (15 oz) black beans, rinsed and drained
- 1/2 cup of corn kernels (fresh or frozen)
- 1/2 cup of diced tomatoes
- 1 small onion, diced
- 2 garlic cloves, minced
- 1 teaspoon ground cumin
- 1/2 teaspoon smoked paprika
- Salt and pepper to taste
- 2 tablespoons olive oil
- Fresh cilantro, chopped (optional for garnish)
- 1/4 cup of avocado or vegan cheese (optional for topping)

Instructions

1. Preheat the oven to 375°F (190° C). Lightly butter a baking dish and leave aside.
2. In a large skillet, warm 1 tablespoon olive oil over medium heat. Sauté the diced onion for 4-5 minutes, until softened.
3. Add the garlic, cumin, smoked paprika and sauté for another minute.
4. Add the cooked quinoa, black beans, corn, and chopped tomatoes to the pan. Stir well and season with salt and pepper to taste. Cook for a further 2-3 minutes to blend the flavors.
5. Drizzle 1 tablespoon olive oil into each bell pepper and season liberally with salt.
6. Stuff each bell pepper with the quinoa mixture, carefully pushing it down to fill it.
7. Place the filled peppers upright in the prepared baking dish. Cover with foil and bake for 30–35 minutes or until the peppers are soft.
8. If using, remove the foil in the last 5 minutes of roasting and top each pepper with avocado slices or vegan cheese.
9. Garnish with fresh cilantro and serve warm.

Nutrition Information (Per Serving):

Calories: 320 Protein: 10g Carbohydrates: 45g Fat: 10g Fiber: 12g Sodium: 400mg Sugar: 7g

Eggplant and Lentil Bolognese

Prep Time: 15 minutes **Cook Time:** 35 minutes **Serving: 4**

Ingredients

- 1 large eggplant, diced
- 1 cup of dried lentils (green or brown), rinsed
- 2 tablespoons olive oil
- 1 onion, chopped
- 2 garlic cloves, minced
- 1 carrot, diced
- 2 celery stalks, diced
- 1 can (14.5 oz) diced tomatoes
- 1 tablespoon tomato paste
- 1 teaspoon dried oregano
- 1 teaspoon dried basil
- 1/2 teaspoon smoked paprika (optional)
- 4 cups of vegetable broth (or water)
- Salt and pepper to taste
- Fresh basil for garnish (optional)
- Cooked pasta of your choice (whole wheat, gluten-free, etc.)

Instructions

1. In a large saucepan, heat 1 tablespoon olive oil over medium heat. Cook the diced eggplant for 5-7 minutes, until cooked and gently browned. Remove from the saucepan and put aside.
2. In the same saucepan, combine the remaining tablespoon of olive oil. Sauté the chopped onion, carrot, and celery for 4-5 minutes, until softened.
3. Cook for another minute, stirring in the garlic, oregano, basil, and smoked paprika (if using), until aromatic.
4. Combine the lentils, diced tomatoes, tomato paste, and vegetable broth. Bring the mixture to a boil, then decrease the heat and cook for 20-25 minutes or until the lentils are cooked.
5. Return the cooked eggplant to the saucepan and stir until combined. Season with salt and pepper to taste. Simmer for a further 5 minutes to let the flavors mingle.
6. Serve the bolognese over cooked pasta, topped with fresh basil if preferred.

Nutrition Information (Per Serving):

Calories: 320 Protein: 15g Carbohydrates: 50g Fat: 8g Fiber: 15g Sodium: 400mg Sugar: 10g

Spicy Tofu Stir-Fry with Vegetables

Prep Time: 10 minutes **Cook Time:** 15 minutes **Serving: 4**

Ingredients

- 1 block (14 oz) firm tofu, pressed and cubed
- 2 tablespoons olive oil or sesame oil
- 1 red bell pepper, sliced
- 1 yellow bell pepper, sliced
- 1 zucchini, sliced
- 1 carrot, julienned
- 2 cups of broccoli florets
- 3 garlic cloves, minced
- 1 tablespoon fresh ginger, grated
- 1/4 cup of low-sodium soy sauce (or tamari for gluten-free)
- 1 tablespoon sriracha or chili garlic sauce
- 1 tablespoon rice vinegar
- 1 teaspoon sesame oil
- 1 tablespoon sesame seeds
- Green onions, chopped

Instructions

1. Heat 1 tablespoon olive oil in a large pan or wok over medium-high heat. Cook the cubed tofu for 5-7 minutes, stirring periodically, until golden brown and crispy. Remove from the skillet and put aside.
2. In the same skillet, heat the remaining 1 tablespoon oil. Sauté the garlic and ginger for 1 minute, until aromatic.
3. Add the bell peppers, zucchini, carrots, and broccoli to the skillet. Stir-fry the veggies for 4-5 minutes until soft yet crisp.
4. In a small mixing bowl, combine the soy sauce, sriracha or chili garlic sauce, rice vinegar, and sesame oil (if using). Pour the sauce over the veggies, stirring to coat.
5. Return the tofu to the skillet and mix everything. Cook for another 2 minutes until heated through.
6. Serve the stir-fry hot, topped with sesame seeds and green onions as desired.

Nutrition Information (Per Serving):

Calories: 270 Protein: 14g Carbohydrates: 20g Fat: 15g Fiber: 5g Sodium: 600mg Sugar: 5g

Butternut Squash Risotto

Prep Time: 10 minutes **Cook Time:** 35-40 minutes **Serving: 4**

Ingredients

- 1 cup of Arborio rice
- 2 tablespoons olive oil
- 1 small onion, finely chopped
- 2 garlic cloves, minced
- 2 cups of butternut squash, peeled and diced
- 4 cups of vegetable broth, warmed
- 1/2 cup of dry white wine (optional)
- 1/4 cup of nutritional yeast
- 1/2 teaspoon ground nutmeg
- Salt and pepper to taste
- Fresh parsley for garnish (optional)

Instructions

1. In a large pot, heat 1 tablespoon olive oil over medium heat. Cook the chopped butternut squash for 8-10 minutes or until softened and faintly caramelized. Remove from the saucepan and put aside.
2. In the same saucepan, combine the remaining tablespoon of olive oil. Sauté the onion and garlic for 3-4 minutes, until softened.
3. Stir in the Arborio rice and heat for 1-2 minutes, until gently toasted.
4. Pour in the white wine (if using) and simmer for 1-2 minutes, stirring regularly until absorbed.
5. Add the hot vegetable broth, one ladleful at a time, while stirring regularly. Allow each ladleful of broth to soak before adding another. Continue cooking for approximately 20-25 minutes or until the rice is creamy and fully cooked.
6. Add the cooked butternut squash to the risotto and the nutritional yeast (or Parmesan), nutmeg, salt, and pepper. Cook for another 2-3 minutes until heated through.
7. Remove from heat, and if preferred, garnish with fresh parsley. Serve immediately.

Nutrition Information (Per Serving):

Calories: 340 Protein: 8g Carbohydrates: 60g Fat: 8g Fiber: 4g Sodium: 500mg Sugar: 4g

Chickpea and Sweet Potato Stew

Prep Time: 10 minutes **Cook Time:** 25-30 minutes **Serving: 4**

Ingredients

- 1 tablespoon olive oil
- 1 onion, chopped
- 2 garlic cloves, minced
- 1 tablespoon fresh ginger, grated
- 1 medium sweet potato, peeled and diced
- 1 can (15 oz) chickpeas, rinsed and drained
- 1 can (14.5 oz) diced tomatoes
- 4 cups of vegetable broth
- 1 teaspoon ground cumin
- 1/2 teaspoon ground turmeric
- 1/4 teaspoon cinnamon (optional)
- Salt and pepper to taste
- 2 cups of fresh spinach, chopped
- Fresh cilantro for garnish (optional)

Instructions

1. In a large saucepan, warm the olive oil over medium heat. Sauté the chopped onion for 4-5 minutes, until softened.
2. Add the garlic and ginger and simmer for another minute or until fragrant.
3. Mix in the chopped sweet potato, chickpeas, tomatoes, vegetable broth, cumin, turmeric, cinnamon (if using), salt, and pepper. Bring the mixture to a boil, then decrease heat and let it simmer for 20-25 minutes, or until the sweet potatoes are cooked.
4. Add the chopped spinach and simmer for 2-3 minutes or until wilted.
5. Taste and adjust the seasoning as required. Garnish with fresh cilantro and serve warm.

Nutrition Information (Per Serving):

Calories: 320 Protein: 9g Carbohydrates: 55g Fat: 8g Fiber: 11g Sodium: 500mg Sugar: 10g

Zucchini Lasagna with Cashew Cheese

Prep Time: 20 minutes **Cook Time:** 40 minutes **Serving: 4**

Ingredients

- For the Zucchini Lasagna:
- 3 medium zucchinis, sliced lengthwise into thin strips
- 1 jar (24 oz) marinara sauce (sugar-free)
- 1 tablespoon olive oil
- 1 onion, chopped
- 3 garlic cloves, minced
- 1 cup of fresh spinach, chopped
- Salt and pepper to taste
- For the Cashew Cheese:
- 1 cup of raw cashews, soaked in water for at least 2 hours
- 1/4 cup of nutritional yeast
- 1 tablespoon lemon juice
- 1 garlic clove
- 1/4 cup of water (adjust for desired consistency)
- Salt and pepper to taste

Instructions

1. Drain the cashews and transfer them to a blender or food processor with the nutritional yeast, lemon juice, garlic, water, salt, and pepper.
2. Blend until smooth and creamy, adding more water for a spreadable consistency. Set aside.
3. Preheat the oven to 375° Fahrenheit (190° Celsius).
4. Heat the olive oil in a pan over medium heat. Sauté the chopped onion and garlic for 4-5 minutes, until softened.
5. Add the chopped spinach and simmer for 1-2 minutes or until wilted. Season with salt and pepper then put away.
6. Cover the bottom of a baking dish with a thin coating of marinara sauce. Layer the zucchini strips on the sauce, then add the sautéed veggies and cashew cheese.
7. Repeat the layers (marinara sauce, zucchini strips, sautéed veggies, cashew cheese) until all ingredients are utilized, followed by a layer of zucchini and marinara sauce on top.
8. Cover the lasagna with foil and bake for 30 minutes. Remove the cover and continue baking for 10 minutes until the top is bubbling and the zucchini is soft.

9. Let the lasagna rest for 5 minutes before serving. If desired, garnish with fresh herbs such as basil or parsley.

Nutrition Information (Per Serving):

Calories: 350 Protein: 12g Carbohydrates: 30g Fat: 20g Fiber: 7g Sodium: 550mg Sugar: 10g

Vegan Cauliflower Tacos

Prep Time: 15 minutes **Cook Time:** 25 minutes **Serve:** 4 servings

Ingredients

- 1 medium head cauliflower, chopped into small florets
- 2 tbsp olive oil
- 1 tsp ground cumin
- 1 tsp smoked paprika
- 1/2 tsp turmeric powder
- 1/2 tsp garlic powder
- Salt and pepper to taste
- 8 small corn tortillas (gluten-free if necessary)
- 1 cup of shredded lettuce
- 1/2 cup of diced tomatoes
- 1/2 cup of diced avocado
- 1/4 cup of chopped fresh cilantro
- 1/4 cup of vegan sour cream (optional)

Instructions

1. Preheat the oven to 400 °F (200 °C). Line a baking sheet with parchment paper.
2. Combine the cauliflower florets, olive oil, cumin, smoked paprika, turmeric, garlic powder, salt, and pepper in a large mixing bowl until equally covered.
3. Spread the cauliflower evenly on the prepared baking sheet, then roast for 20-25 minutes or until golden and crispy, tossing halfway through.
4. While the cauliflower is roasting, cook the corn tortillas in a dry pan over medium heat for approximately 1 minute on each side.
5. Place roasted cauliflower in each tortilla, then top with shredded lettuce, chopped tomatoes, avocado, and fresh cilantro.
6. Optional: Top with a spoonful of vegan sour cream for added richness.
7. Serve immediately and enjoy!

Nutrition Information (per serving):

Calories: 210 Protein: 5g Fat: 11g Carbohydrates: 23g Fiber: 7g Sugar: 3g Sodium: 210mg

Quinoa Stuffed Tomatoes

Prep Time: 15 minutes **Cook Time:** 30 minutes **Serve:** 4 servings

Ingredients

- 4 large ripe tomatoes
- 1 cup of cooked quinoa
- 1/4 cup of finely chopped red bell pepper
- 1/4 cup of finely chopped zucchini
- 2 tbsp finely chopped red onion
- 2 tbsp fresh parsley, chopped
- 1 tbsp fresh basil, chopped
- 1 tbsp olive oil
- 1/4 tsp turmeric powder
- Salt and pepper to taste
- 1 tbsp lemon juice
- 2 tbsp vegan Parmesan (optional)

Instructions

1. Preheat the oven to 375° Fahrenheit (190° Celsius). Grease a baking dish gently with olive oil.
2. Slice off the tops of the tomatoes and scoop out the pulp and seeds with a spoon, taking care not to damage the skin. Set aside the tomato shells, then cut the tomato pulp.
3. Add the cooked quinoa, diced red bell pepper, zucchini, red onion, parsley, basil, olive oil, turmeric powder, salt, pepper, and lemon juice in a mixing bowl. Mix well to mix.
4. Combine the diced tomato pulp with the quinoa mixture.
5. Stuff each tomato with the quinoa mixture and put in a greased baking dish.
6. If desired, sprinkle vegan Parmesan over each filled tomato.
7. Bake for 25 to 30 minutes or until the tomatoes are soft and the tops are golden.
8. Allow to cool slightly before serving.

Nutrition Information (per serving):

Calories: 180 Protein: 5g Fat: 7g Carbohydrates: 24g Fiber: 4g Sugar: 5g Sodium: 140mg

Moroccan Vegetable Tagine

Prep Time: 20 minutes **Cook Time:** 40 minutes **Serve:** 4 servings

Ingredients

- 1 tbsp olive oil
- 1 medium onion, diced
- 3 garlic cloves, minced
- 2 medium carrots, sliced
- 1 small zucchini, chopped
- 1 small eggplant, chopped
- 1 cup of butternut squash, peeled and cubed
- 1 can (14.5 oz) diced tomatoes, no salt added
- 1 can (15 oz) chickpeas, drained and rinsed
- 1/2 cup of vegetable broth (low sodium)
- 1/2 tsp ground cumin
- 1/2 tsp ground cinnamon
- 1/2 tsp ground turmeric
- 1/4 tsp ground ginger
- 1/4 tsp smoked paprika
- Salt and pepper to taste
- 1/4 cup of raisins or chopped dried apricots
- 2 tbsp fresh parsley or cilantro, chopped (for garnish)
- 1/2 cup of cooked quinoa (optional for serving)

Instructions

1. Heat the olive oil in a large saucepan or tagine over medium heat. Sauté the diced onion for 3-4 minutes, until softened.
2. Combine the garlic, carrots, zucchini, eggplant, and butternut squash. Cook for 5–6 minutes, stirring periodically.
3. Combine the chopped tomatoes, chickpeas, and vegetable broth. Combine the cumin, cinnamon, turmeric, ginger, smoked paprika, salt, and pepper.
4. Bring the mixture to a boil, decrease heat to low, cover, and cook for 25-30 minutes or until the veggies are soft.
5. Stir in the raisins or chopped dried apricots in the final 5 minutes of simmering to soften and give sweetness.
6. Taste and adjust spices as needed.
7. Garnish with fresh parsley or cilantro before serving. If preferred, serve the tagine over cooked quinoa.

Nutrition Information (per serving):

Calories: 250 Protein: 7g Fat: 7g Carbohydrates: 42g Fiber: 9g Sugar: 13g Sodium: 260mg

Vegan Eggplant Parmesan

Prep Time: 20 minutes **Cook Time:** 40 minutes **Serve:** 4 servings

Ingredients

- 1 large eggplant, sliced into 1/2-inch rounds
- 1 tsp salt (for sweating the eggplant)
- 1 cup of almond flour
- 1/2 cup of nutritional yeast
- 1/2 tsp dried oregano
- 1/2 tsp dried basil
- 1/2 tsp garlic powder
- 1/4 tsp turmeric powder
- 1/4 cup of unsweetened almond milk
- 2 cups of marinara sauce (low sodium)
- 1/2 cup of vegan mozzarella cheese (optional)
- 1 tbsp olive oil (for greasing the baking sheet)
- Fresh basil, chopped (for garnish)

Instructions

1. Preheat the oven to 400 °F (200 °C). Line a baking sheet with parchment paper and gently coat it with olive oil.
2. Lay the eggplant slices on a chopping board and season with salt on both sides. Allow them to sit for 15-20 minutes to sweat off any extra moisture. Dry them with a paper towel.
3. Mix the almond flour, nutritional yeast, dried oregano, dried basil, garlic powder, and turmeric in a bowl.
4. Pour the almond milk into a separate, small bowl.
5. Dip each eggplant slice in almond milk, then coat it with the almond flour. Place the coated slices on the prepared baking sheet.
6. Bake the eggplant slices for 20 minutes, turning halfway, until golden and crispy.
7. Remove the baking sheet from the oven. Spread a small amount of marinara sauce over each eggplant slice, then top with vegan mozzarella if preferred.

8. Return the baking sheet to the oven and cook for 15-20 minutes or until the cheese is melted and bubbling.
9. Before serving, garnish with freshly chopped basil.

Nutrition Information (per serving):

Calories: 220 Protein: 7g Fat: 13g Carbohydrates: 21g Fiber: 8g Sugar: 7g Sodium: 350mg

Roasted Vegetable Quinoa Bowl

Prep Time: 15 minutes **Cook Time:** 30 minutes **Serve:** 4 servings

Ingredients

- 1 cup of quinoa, rinsed
- 2 cups of water
- 1 medium zucchini, chopped
- 1 red bell pepper, chopped
- 1 yellow bell pepper, chopped
- 1 small red onion, chopped
- 1 cup of cherry tomatoes
- 2 tbsp olive oil
- 1 tsp dried oregano
- 1/2 tsp ground turmeric
- Salt and pepper to taste
- 1/4 cup of chopped fresh parsley
- 1 tbsp lemon juice

Instructions

1. Preheat the oven to 400 °F (200 °C). Line a baking sheet with parchment paper.
2. In a medium saucepan, bring 2 cups of water to a boil. Add the rinsed quinoa, lower heat to low, cover, and simmer for 15 minutes, or until the quinoa is cooked and the water has been absorbed. Fluff with a fork, then put aside.
3. While the quinoa cooks, arrange the zucchini, bell peppers, red onion, and cherry tomatoes on the prepared baking sheet.
4. Drizzle the veggies with olive oil, then season with dried oregano, turmeric, salt, and pepper. Toss to coat evenly.
5. Roast the veggies in a warm oven for 20-25 minutes or until soft and faintly caramelized.

6. In a large bowl, combine the cooked quinoa with the roasted veggies. Stir in the chopped parsley and lemon juice.
7. Serve warm or at room temperature.

Nutrition Information (per serving):

Calories: 240 Protein: 6g Fat: 10g Carbohydrates: 32g Fiber: 5g Sugar: 5g Sodium: 180mg

Vegan Vegetable Paella

Prep Time: 15 minutes **Cook Time:** 35 minutes **Serve:** 4 servings

Ingredients

- 1 tbsp olive oil
- 1 medium onion, finely chopped
- 3 garlic cloves, minced
- 1 red bell pepper, sliced
- 1 yellow bell pepper, sliced
- 1 medium zucchini, chopped
- 1 cup of green beans, trimmed
- 1 1/2 cups of Arborio rice or short-grain rice
- 1 tsp smoked paprika
- 1/2 tsp ground turmeric
- 1/2 tsp sweet paprika
- 1/4 tsp saffron threads (optional)
- 1 can (14.5 oz) diced tomatoes, no salt added
- 3 cups of vegetable broth (low sodium)
- 1 cup of frozen peas
- Salt and pepper to taste
- 1/4 cup of chopped fresh parsley
- Lemon wedges for serving

Instructions:

1. Heat the olive oil in a large skillet or paella pan over medium heat. Sauté the chopped onion for 3-4 minutes, until softened.
2. Combine the minced garlic, red and yellow bell peppers, zucchini, and green beans. Cook for 5 more minutes, stirring periodically.

3. Add the Arborio rice to the pan and toss to coat with the vegetable mixture. Cook for 2-3 minutes, until the rice has toasted somewhat.
4. Combine the smoked paprika, turmeric, sweet paprika, and saffron (if using). Stir in the diced tomatoes and veggie broth until well combined.
5. Bring the mixture to a boil, then lower the heat. Cover and cook for 20-25 minutes until the rice is cooked and the liquid has been absorbed.
6. Stir in the frozen peas in the final 5 minutes of cooking. Season with salt and pepper to taste.
7. Remove from the heat and allow the paella to settle for 5 minutes. Garnish with fresh parsley and serve with lemon wedges on the side.

Nutrition Information (per serving):

Calories: 280 Protein: 6g Fat: 7g Carbohydrates: 48g Fiber: 7g Sugar: 7g Sodium: 240mg

CHAPTER 6: POULTRY AND MEAT

Grilled Chicken with Turmeric and Lime

Prep Time: 15 minutes **Cook Time:** 20 minutes **Serve:** 4 servings

Ingredients

- 4 boneless, skinless chicken breasts
- 2 tbsp olive oil
- 1 tsp ground turmeric
- 1/2 tsp ground cumin
- 1/2 tsp smoked paprika
- 1/4 tsp black pepper
- 1/4 tsp salt
- Juice of 2 limes
- 2 garlic cloves, minced
- 1 tbsp fresh cilantro, chopped (for garnish)

Instructions

1. In a small mixing bowl, combine the olive oil, turmeric, cumin, smoked paprika, black pepper, salt, lime juice, and chopped garlic to make the marinade.
2. Place the chicken breasts in a shallow dish or a sealable plastic bag. Pour the marinade over the chicken, ensuring each piece is well covered. Cover and chill for at least 30 minutes.
3. Preheat the grill to medium-high heat. Grill the chicken breasts on each side for 5-6 minutes, or until the internal temperature reaches 165°F (74°C) and the chicken is well cooked.
4. Remove the chicken from the grill and rest for 5 minutes.
5. Garnish with chopped cilantro before serving.

Nutrition Information (per serving):

Calories: 220 Protein: 27g Fat: 11g Carbohydrates: 2g Fiber: 1g Sugar: 0g Sodium: 230mg

Roasted Chicken with Garlic and Thyme

Prep Time: 15 minutes **Cook Time:** 1 hour 15 minutes **Serve:** 4 servings

Ingredients

- 1 whole chicken (about 4 lbs)
- 2 tbsp olive oil
- 6 garlic cloves, minced
- 2 tbsp fresh thyme leaves
- 1 tsp ground turmeric
- 1/2 tsp black pepper
- 1/2 tsp salt
- 1 lemon, halved
- 1 medium onion, quartered
- 2 carrots, chopped
- 1 cup of low-sodium chicken broth

Instructions

1. Preheat the oven to 375° Fahrenheit (190° Celsius). Place a roasting rack in a roasting pan.
2. In a small bowl, combine olive oil, minced garlic, thyme, turmeric, black pepper, and salt.
3. Rub the spice mixture all over the chicken, coating the skin evenly. Insert the lemon halves into the cavity of the bird.
4. Place the onion quarters and sliced carrots in a roasting pan. Place the seasoned chicken on the roasting rack above the veggies.
5. Pour chicken stock into the roasting pan to keep the veggies wet while cooking.
6. Roast the chicken in a preheated oven for approximately 1 hour and 15 minutes, or until the internal temperature reaches 165°F (74°C) and the juices are clear. Baste the chicken with pan juices from time to time.
7. Remove the chicken from the oven and rest for 10 minutes before carving.
8. Serve with roasted veggies and, if preferred, garnish with more thyme.

Nutrition Information (per serving):

Calories: 350 Protein: 30g Fat: 23g Carbohydrates: 7g Fiber: 2g Sugar: 3g Sodium: 260mg

Chicken and Sweet Potato Stir-Fry

Prep Time: 15 minutes **Cook Time:** 25 minutes **Serve:** 4 servings

Ingredients

- 2 tbsp olive oil
- 2 boneless, skinless chicken breasts cut into bite-sized pieces
- 1 medium sweet potato, peeled and cut into small cubes
- 1 red bell pepper, sliced
- 1 small onion, sliced
- 2 garlic cloves, minced
- 1/2 tsp ground turmeric
- 1/2 tsp ground ginger
- 1/4 tsp black pepper
- 1/4 tsp salt
- 2 tbsp low-sodium soy sauce
- 1 tbsp lemon juice
- 2 tbsp fresh parsley, chopped (for garnish)

Instructions

1. Heat 1 tablespoon olive oil in a large pan or wok over medium heat. Cook the diced sweet potato for 5-7 minutes, stirring regularly, until slightly soft. Remove from the skillet and put aside.
2. Warm the remaining tablespoon of olive oil over medium-high heat in the same skillet. Cook the chicken pieces for 5-6 minutes until browned and cooked.
3. Add the chopped onion, red bell pepper, and minced garlic to the pan. Cook for 4-5 minutes, until the veggies have softened.
4. Mix the cooked sweet potatoes, turmeric, ground ginger, black pepper, and salt. Cook for 2-3 minutes, stirring to incorporate all the flavors.
5. Add the low-sodium soy sauce and lemon juice, stirring to coat the chicken and veggies evenly. Cook for another 1–2 minutes.
6. Remove from the heat and sprinkle with fresh parsley before serving.

Nutrition Information (per serving):

Calories: 260 Protein: 23g Fat: 11g Carbohydrates: 18g Fiber: 3g Sugar: 5g Sodium: 310mg

Lemon Rosemary Roasted Turkey

Prep Time: 20 minutes **Cook Time:** 2 hours 30 minutes **Serve:** 8 servings

Ingredients

- 1 whole turkey breast (about 5 lbs)
- 3 tbsp olive oil
- 2 tbsp fresh rosemary, chopped
- 1 tbsp fresh thyme, chopped
- 1 tsp ground turmeric
- 4 garlic cloves, minced
- 1 tsp black pepper
- 1/2 tsp salt
- Juice of 2 lemons
- Zest of 1 lemon
- 1 lemon, sliced
- 1 cup of low-sodium chicken broth

Instructions

1. To make the marinade, combine olive oil, chopped rosemary, thyme, turmeric, minced garlic, black pepper, salt, lemon juice, and lemon zest in a small mixing dish.
2. Rub the marinade all over the turkey breast, coating it evenly. Cover and chill for at least 2 hours to enable the flavors to combine.
3. Preheat the oven to 350° Fahrenheit (175° Celsius). Place the turkey breast in a roasting pan and top with lemon wedges.
4. Pour chicken stock into the bottom of the roasting pan to keep the turkey wet while cooking.
5. Cook the turkey in the oven for 2 to 2 1/2 hours or until the internal temperature reaches 165°F (74°C). Baste the turkey with pan juices from time to time.
6. Take the turkey out of the oven and rest for 10-15 minutes before slicing.
7. Serve with pan juices; garnish with more fresh rosemary if desired.

Nutrition Information (per serving):

Calories: 290 Protein: 46g Fat: 10g Carbohydrates: 3g Sugar: 1g Sodium: 260mg

Grilled Chicken Skewers with Veggies

Prep Time: 20 minutes **Cook Time:** 15 minutes **Serve:** 4 servings

Ingredients

- 2 boneless, skinless chicken breasts cut into 1-inch cubes
- 1 red bell pepper, cut into 1-inch pieces
- 1 yellow bell pepper, cut into 1-inch pieces
- 1 zucchini, sliced into rounds
- 1 red onion, cut into chunks
- 2 tbsp olive oil
- Juice of 1 lemon
- 1 tsp ground turmeric
- 1/2 tsp ground cumin
- 1/2 tsp smoked paprika
- 1/4 tsp black pepper
- 1/4 tsp salt
- 2 garlic cloves, minced
- Fresh parsley, chopped (for garnish)

Instructions

1. In a large mixing bowl, combine the olive oil, lemon juice, turmeric, cumin, smoked paprika, black pepper, salt, and chopped garlic to make the marinade.
2. Add the chicken cubes to the marinade, ensuring they're completely covered. Cover and chill for at least 30 minutes.
3. Preheat the grill to medium-high heat. Soak wooden skewers in water for 15 minutes before use to avoid scorching.
4. Thread marinated chicken, bell peppers, zucchini, and red onion onto skewers, alternating between the veggies and the chicken.
5. Grill the skewers for 10-15 minutes, rotating regularly, until the chicken is well cooked and the veggies are soft and slightly browned.
6. Remove off the grill and let it cool for a few minutes. Before serving, garnish with finely chopped fresh parsley.

Nutrition Information (per serving):

Calories: 220 Protein: 23g Fat: 10g Carbohydrates: 8g Fiber: 2g Sugar: 4g Sodium: 230mg

Balsamic Glazed Chicken Thighs

Prep Time: 10 minutes **Cook Time:** 30 minutes **Serve:** 4 servings

Ingredients

- 8 bone-in, skinless chicken thighs
- 1/4 cup of balsamic vinegar
- 2 tbsp olive oil
- 1 tbsp honey
- 3 garlic cloves, minced
- 1 tsp dried thyme
- 1/2 tsp ground turmeric
- 1/4 tsp black pepper
- 1/4 tsp salt
- 1 tbsp chopped fresh parsley (for garnish)

Instructions

1. Mix the balsamic vinegar, olive oil, honey, minced garlic, dried thyme, turmeric, black pepper, and salt in a large mixing bowl to make the marinade.
2. Add the chicken thighs to the bowl, ensuring they are fully covered in the marinade. Cover and chill for at least 30 minutes to enable the flavors to combine.
3. Preheat the oven to 400 °F (200 °C). Put the marinated chicken thighs onto a baking dish.
4. Pour any leftover marinade over the chicken and bake for 25-30 minutes or until thoroughly cooked with an internal temperature of 165°F (74°C).
5. Turn on the broiler for 2-3 minutes to caramelize the glaze.
6. Take the chicken out of the oven and rest for a few minutes. Before serving, garnish with finely chopped fresh parsley.

Nutrition Information (per serving):

Calories: 270 Protein: 24g Fat: 14g Carbohydrates: 8g Fiber: 0g Sugar: 6g Sodium: 260mg

Chicken and Zucchini Lettuce Wraps

Prep Time: 15 minutes **Cook Time:** 15 minutes **Serve:** 4 servings

Ingredients

- 2 tbsp olive oil
- 1 lb ground chicken
- 1 small onion, finely chopped
- 2 garlic cloves, minced
- 1 medium zucchini, grated
- 1 red bell pepper, finely chopped
- 1/2 tsp ground turmeric
- 1/2 tsp ground cumin
- 1/4 tsp black pepper
- 1/4 tsp salt
- 2 tbsp low-sodium soy sauce (or tamari for gluten-free)
- 1 tbsp fresh lime juice
- 8 large lettuce leaves (e.g., butter or romaine lettuce)
- 2 tbsp chopped fresh cilantro (for garnish)

Instructions

1. Heat the olive oil in a large pan over medium heat. Add the chopped onion and simmer for 3-4 minutes or until tender.
2. Add the minced garlic and simmer for another minute.
3. Add the ground chicken and simmer for 5-6 minutes, breaking it up with a spatula until browned and cooked.
4. Add the grated zucchini and red bell pepper to the skillet. Cook for a further 3-4 minutes until the veggies are soft.
5. Combine the turmeric, cumin, black pepper, salt, soy sauce, and lime juice. Mix thoroughly and heat for a further 1-2 minutes.
6. Remove from the heat and allow the mixture to cool somewhat.
7. Before serving, spoon the chicken and vegetable mixture onto the lettuce leaves and top with chopped fresh cilantro.

Nutrition Information (per serving):

Calories: 200 Protein: 23g Fat: 10g Carbohydrates: 7g Fiber: 2g Sugar: 3g Sodium: 260mg

Slow-cooked beef and Sweet Potato Stew

Prep Time: 20 minutes **Cook Time:** 6-8 hours **Serve:** 6 servings

Ingredients

- 1 1/2 lbs beef stew meat, cut into 1-inch cubes
- 2 tbsp olive oil
- 1 medium onion, chopped
- 3 garlic cloves, minced
- 2 medium sweet potatoes, peeled and cut into 1-inch cubes
- 2 large carrots, sliced
- 1 red bell pepper, chopped
- 1 tsp ground turmeric
- 1 tsp smoked paprika
- 1/2 tsp ground cumin
- 1/2 tsp dried thyme
- 1/2 tsp black pepper
- 1/2 tsp salt
- 3 cups of low-sodium beef broth
- 1 tbsp apple cider vinegar
- 1 bay leaf
- 2 tbsp chopped fresh parsley (for garnish)

Instructions

1. Heat 1 tablespoon olive oil in a large pan over medium-high heat. Add the meat cubes and cook for 3-4 minutes or until browned on both sides. Transfer the meat to the slow cooker.
2. Heat the remaining olive oil in the same skillet and cook the chopped onion for 3-4 minutes or until softened. Add the minced garlic and simmer for another minute.
3. Place the onion and garlic in the slow cooker, along with the sweet potatoes, carrots, and red bell peppers.
4. Combine the turmeric, smoked paprika, cumin, thyme, black pepper, and salt.
5. Pour the beef broth and apple cider vinegar, then add the bay leaf. Stir everything together.
6. Cover and simmer on low for 6-8 hours or until the meat is tender and the veggies are fully cooked.
7. Remove the bay leaf, add the chopped fresh parsley, and serve warm.

Nutrition Information (per serving):

Calories: 280 Protein: 25g Fat: 11g Carbohydrates: 20g Fiber: 4g Sugar: 6g Sodium: 310mg

Grilled Turkey Burgers with Avocado

Prep Time: 15 minutes **Cook Time:** 15 minutes **Serve:** 4 servings

Ingredients

- 1 lb ground turkey
- 1/2 small onion, finely chopped
- 2 garlic cloves, minced
- 1/2 tsp ground turmeric
- 1/2 tsp ground cumin
- 1/4 tsp black pepper
- 1/4 tsp salt
- 1 tbsp fresh parsley, chopped
- 1 tbsp olive oil
- 1 ripe avocado, sliced
- 4 whole wheat burger buns (or lettuce wraps for a low-carb option)
- 4 lettuce leaves
- 4 slices of tomato

Instructions

1. Add ground turkey, diced onion, minced garlic, turmeric, cumin, black pepper, salt, and parsley in a large mixing bowl. Mix until well mixed.
2. Divide the ingredients into four equal pieces, shaping each into a patty.
3. Preheat the grill over medium-high heat and brush with olive oil to avoid sticking.
4. Place the turkey patties on the grill for 5-6 minutes on each side or until the internal temperature reaches 165°F (74°C) and the burgers are well cooked.
5. While the burgers cook, toast the buns on the grill for around 1-2 minutes.
6. Make the burgers by putting a lettuce leaf and a piece of tomato on the bottom half of each bun. Top the cooked turkey patty with avocado slices. Put the top bun over the avocado.
7. Serve immediately and enjoy!

Nutrition Information (per serving):

Calories: 320 Protein: 25g Fat: 17g Carbohydrates: 20g Fiber: 5g Sugar: 3g Sodium: 270mg

Herb-Crusted Lamb Chops

Prep Time: 15 minutes

Cook Time: 20 minutes

Serve: 4 servings

Ingredients

- 8 lamb chops (about 1 inch thick)
- 2 tbsp olive oil
- 2 tbsp fresh rosemary, chopped
- 1 tbsp fresh thyme, chopped
- 1 tsp dried oregano
- 1/2 tsp ground turmeric
- 3 garlic cloves, minced
- 1/2 tsp black pepper
- 1/4 tsp salt
- Juice of 1 lemon

Instructions

1. Mix the olive oil, chopped rosemary, thyme, oregano, turmeric, minced garlic, black pepper, salt, and lemon juice in a small mixing bowl to make a marinade.
2. Rub the marinade evenly over the lamb chops, ensuring they are well covered. Cover and chill for at least 30 minutes to enable the flavors to combine.
3. Preheat the grill or grill pan to medium-high temperature.
4. Grill the lamb chops for approximately 3-4 minutes each side for medium-rare, or modify the cooking time to your desired doneness. Use a meat thermometer to ensure the medium-rare internal temperature is at least 145°F (63°C).
5. Remove the lamb chops from the grill and let them rest for 5 minutes before serving.

Nutrition Information (per serving):

Calories: 340 Protein: 25g Fat: 25g Carbohydrates: 3g Fiber: 1g Sugar: 0g Sodium: 180mg

Beef and Barley Soup

Prep Time: 20 minutes **Cook Time:** 1 hour 30 minutes **Serve:** 6 servings

Ingredients

- 1 tbsp olive oil
- 1 lb beef stew meat, cut into 1-inch cubes
- 1 medium onion, chopped
- 3 garlic cloves, minced
- 2 medium carrots, sliced
- 2 celery stalks, chopped
- 1 cup of diced tomatoes, no salt added
- 1/2 cup of pearl barley
- 1 tsp ground turmeric
- 1/2 tsp dried thyme
- 1/2 tsp ground black pepper
- 1/2 tsp salt
- 6 cups of low-sodium beef broth
- 1 bay leaf
- 2 tbsp chopped fresh parsley (for garnish)

Instructions

1. Heat the olive oil in a large saucepan over medium-high heat. Cook the meat cubes for 4-5 minutes until browned on both sides.
2. Add the chopped onions, carrots, and celery to the saucepan. Cook the veggies for 5-6 minutes, stirring periodically until tender.
3. Stir in the minced garlic and simmer for another minute.
4. Combine the chopped tomatoes, pearl barley, turmeric, dried thyme, black pepper, and salt. Stir to mix.
5. Pour in the beef broth, then add the bay leaf. Bring the mixture to a boil, then lower the heat. Cover and simmer for 1 hour and 15 minutes until the meat is soft and the barley is done.
6. Before serving, remove the bay leaf and add some chopped fresh parsley.

Nutrition Information (per serving):

Calories: 250 Protein: 20g Fat: 10g Carbohydrates: 22g Fiber: 4g Sugar: 3g Sodium: 320mg

Chicken Stir-Fry with Bell Peppers

Prep Time: 15 minutes **Cook Time:** 15 minutes **Serve:** 4 servings

Ingredients

- 2 tbsp olive oil
- 2 boneless, skinless chicken breasts, thinly sliced
- 1 red bell pepper, thinly sliced
- 1 yellow bell pepper, thinly sliced
- 1 green bell pepper, thinly sliced
- 1 small onion, thinly sliced
- 2 garlic cloves, minced
- 1/2 tsp ground turmeric
- 1/2 tsp ground ginger
- 1/4 tsp black pepper
- 1/4 tsp salt
- 2 tbsp low-sodium soy sauce (or tamari for gluten-free)
- 1 tbsp fresh lemon juice
- 1 tbsp chopped fresh cilantro (for garnish)

Instructions

1. Heat 1 tablespoon olive oil in a large pan or wok over medium-high heat. Add the sliced chicken and heat for 5-6 minutes or until browned and done. Remove the chicken from the skillet and put it aside.
2. In the same skillet, heat the remaining tablespoon of olive oil. Combine the cut bell peppers, onion, and minced garlic. Stir-fry for 5-6 minutes until the veggies are soft and crisp.
3. Return cooked chicken to the skillet. Combine the turmeric, ground ginger, black pepper, salt, soy sauce, and lemon juice. Cook for another 2-3 minutes, until everything is well mixed and cooked.
4. Garnish with chopped fresh cilantro before serving.

Nutrition Information (per serving):

Calories: 230 Protein: 23g Fat: 11g Carbohydrates: 10g Fiber: 3g Sugar: 4g Sodium: 280mg

Turkey and Zucchini Patties

Prep Time: 15 minutes **Cook Time:** 15 minutes **Serve:** 4 servings

Ingredients

- 1 lb ground turkey
- 1 medium zucchini, grated
- 1 small onion, finely chopped
- 2 garlic cloves, minced
- 1/2 tsp ground turmeric
- 1/2 tsp ground cumin
- 1/4 tsp black pepper
- 1/4 tsp salt
- 1/4 cup of fresh parsley, chopped
- 1 tbsp olive oil (for cooking)

Instructions

1. Mix the ground turkey, grated zucchini, diced onion, minced garlic, turmeric, cumin, black pepper, salt, and chopped parsley in a large mixing bowl. Mix until all ingredients are well combined.
2. Divide the ingredients into eight equal parts, shaping each into a patty.
3. Heat the olive oil in a large pan over medium heat. Add the patties and cook for 5-6 minutes on each side or until browned and cooked through, with an internal temperature of 165°F (74°C).
4. Remove the patties from the grill and let them rest for a few minutes before serving.

Nutrition Information (per serving):

Calories: 180 Protein: 24g Fat: 8g Carbohydrates: 4g Fiber: 1g Sugar: 2g Sodium: 220mg

Spiced Turkey and Sweet Potato Hash

Prep Time: 15 minutes **Cook Time:** 20 minutes **Serve:** 4 servings

Ingredients

- 1 tbsp olive oil
- 1 lb ground turkey
- 1 medium sweet potato, peeled and diced into small cubes
- 1 small onion, chopped
- 1 red bell pepper, chopped
- 2 garlic cloves, minced
- 1 tsp ground turmeric
- 1/2 tsp ground cumin
- 1/4 tsp ground cinnamon
- 1/4 tsp black pepper
- 1/4 tsp salt
- 1 tbsp fresh parsley, chopped (for garnish)

Instructions

1. Heat the olive oil in a large pan over medium heat. Cook the cubed sweet potato for 5-6 minutes or until slightly soft.
2. Add the diced onion, red bell pepper, and minced garlic to the skillet. Cook the veggies for 3-4 minutes, stirring regularly, until they soften.
3. Add the ground turkey to the skillet and mix it with a spatula. Cook for 5-6 minutes or until the turkey is browned and well-cooked.
4. Combine the turmeric, cumin, cinnamon, black pepper, and salt. Cook for 2-3 minutes, ensuring all ingredients are combined and cooked completely.
5. Remove from the heat and sprinkle with fresh parsley before serving.

Nutrition Information (per serving):

Calories: 230 Protein: 21g Fat: 10g Carbohydrates: 16g Fiber: 3g Sugar: 5g Sodium: 240mg

Ginger Chicken Lettuce Wraps

Prep Time: 15 minutes **Cook Time:** 15 minutes **Serve:** 4 servings

Ingredients

- 2 tbsp olive oil
- 1 lb ground chicken
- 1 small onion, finely chopped
- 2 garlic cloves, minced
- 1 tbsp fresh ginger, grated
- 1 medium carrot, grated
- 1 red bell pepper, finely chopped
- 1/2 tsp ground turmeric
- 1/4 tsp black pepper
- 1/4 tsp salt
- 2 tbsp low-sodium soy sauce (or tamari for gluten-free)
- 1 tbsp fresh lime juice
- 8 large lettuce leaves (e.g., butter or romaine lettuce)
- 2 tbsp fresh cilantro, chopped (for garnish)

Instructions

1. Heat 1 tablespoon olive oil in a large pan over medium heat. Add the chopped onion and cook for 3-4 minutes or until softened.
2. Cook for a further minute after adding the minced garlic and grated ginger.
3. Add the ground chicken to the pan and heat for 5-6 minutes, breaking it up with a spatula, until browned and thoroughly cooked.
4. Combine the grated carrot, red bell pepper, turmeric, black pepper, and salt. Cook for another 2-3 minutes until the veggies are soft.
5. Stir in the soy sauce and lime juice until well combined. Cook for another minute until the mixture is well heated.
6. Before serving, spoon the chicken mixture onto lettuce leaves and top with chopped cilantro.

Nutrition Information (per serving):

Calories: 180 Protein: 22g Fat: 9g Carbohydrates: 6g Fiber: 2g Sugar: 3g Sodium: 240mg

Slow Cooker Chicken and Carrot Stew

Prep Time: 15 minutes **Cook Time:** 4-6 hours **Serve:** 4 servings

Ingredients

- 1 1/2 lbs boneless, skinless chicken thighs
- 3 medium carrots, peeled and sliced
- 1 medium onion, chopped
- 3 garlic cloves, minced
- 1 tsp ground turmeric
- 1/2 tsp ground cumin
- 1/2 tsp dried thyme
- 1/2 tsp ground black pepper
- 1/2 tsp salt
- 2 cups of low-sodium chicken broth
- 1 tbsp apple cider vinegar
- 2 tbsp chopped fresh parsley (for garnish)

Instructions

1. Add the chicken thighs, sliced carrots, diced onion, and minced garlic to the slow cooker.
2. Sprinkle turmeric, cumin, thyme, black pepper, and salt over the ingredients in the slow cooker.
3. Add the chicken broth and apple cider vinegar. Stir everything until nicely combined.
4. Cover the slow cooker and cook on low for 6 hours or high for 4 hours until the chicken is cooked and easy to shred.
5. Before serving, sprinkle with chopped fresh parsley.

Nutrition Information (per serving):

Calories: 230 Protein: 28g Fat: 9g Carbohydrates: 9g Fiber: 3g Sugar: 4g Sodium: 250mg

Grilled Lamb with Mint Sauce

Prep Time: 20 minutes **Cook Time:** 15 minutes **Serve:** 4 servings

Ingredients

- 8 lamb chops (about 1 inch thick)
- 2 tbsp olive oil
- 2 garlic cloves, minced
- 1 tsp ground turmeric
- 1/2 tsp dried thyme
- 1/4 tsp black pepper
- 1/4 tsp salt
- Juice of 1 lemon
- 1/4 cup of fresh mint leaves, chopped
- 2 tbsp fresh parsley, chopped
- 1 tbsp apple cider vinegar
- 1 tbsp olive oil
- 1 tsp honey
- Juice of 1/2 lemon
- Salt and pepper to taste

Instructions

1. To make the marinade, combine olive oil, minced garlic, turmeric, thyme, black pepper, salt, and lemon juice in a small mixing bowl.
2. Rub the marinade evenly over the lamb chops, ensuring they are well covered. Cover and chill for at least 30 minutes.
3. While the lamb marinates, make the mint sauce. Add the chopped mint, parsley, apple cider vinegar, olive oil, honey, lemon juice, salt, and pepper in a mixing bowl. Mix well and keep aside.
4. Preheat the grill to medium-high heat.
5. Grill the lamb chops for approximately 3-4 minutes each side for medium-rare, or modify the cooking time to your desired doneness. Use a meat thermometer to ensure the medium-rare internal temperature is at least 145°F (63°C).
6. Remove the lamb chops from the grill and let them rest for 5 minutes before serving. Serve the grilled lamb chops with mint sauce on the side.

Nutrition Information (per serving):

Calories: 320 Protein: 24g Fat: 22g Carbohydrates: 5g Fiber: 1g Sugar: 3g Sodium: 180mg

CHAPTER 7: SNACKS

Roasted Chickpeas with Paprika

Prep Time: 5 minutes **Cook Time:** 30 minutes **Serve:** 4 servings

Ingredients

- 1 can (15 oz) chickpeas, drained and rinsed
- 1 tbsp olive oil
- 1 tsp smoked paprika
- 1/2 tsp ground turmeric
- 1/2 tsp garlic powder
- 1/4 tsp black pepper
- 1/4 tsp salt

Instructions

1. Preheat the oven to 400 °F (200 °C). Line a baking sheet with parchment paper.
2. Spread the drained chickpeas on a clean kitchen towel and wipe dry well.
3. Move the chickpeas to a mixing dish. Combine olive oil, smoked paprika, turmeric, garlic powder, black pepper, and salt. Toss chickpeas until evenly coated.
4. Place the chickpeas in a single layer on the prepared baking sheet.
5. Roast the chickpeas in a preheated oven for 25-30 minutes, stirring the pan halfway through, until golden brown and crispy.
6. Allow roasted chickpeas to cool for a few minutes before serving.

Nutrition Information (per serving):

Calories: 110 Protein: 4g Fat: 5g Carbohydrates: 13g Fiber: 4g Sugar: 1g Sodium: 170mg

Almond Butter and Banana Bites

Prep Time: 10 minutes **Cook Time:** None **Serve:** 4 servings

Ingredients

- 2 ripe bananas
- 4 tbsp almond butter
- 2 tbsp chopped almonds
- 1/2 tsp ground cinnamon
- 1/4 tsp ground turmeric (optional)

Instructions

1. Peel the bananas and cut them into half-inch rounds.
2. Spread a tiny quantity of almond butter onto each banana slice.
3. Sprinkle chopped almonds on top of the almond butter.
4. Lightly sprinkle each banana bite with ground cinnamon and turmeric to provide an additional anti-inflammatory kick.
5. Serve immediately or chill for a few minutes if you like them cold.

Nutrition Information (per serving):

Calories: 140 Protein: 3g Fat: 8g Carbohydrates: 16g Fiber: 3g Sugar: 8g Sodium: 2mg

Apple Slices with Almond Butter

Prep Time: 5 minutes

Cook Time: None

Serve: 2 servings

Ingredients

- 1 large apple cored and sliced
- 4 tbsp almond butter
- 1/2 tsp ground cinnamon
- 1 tbsp chopped almonds (optional)

Instructions

1. Place the apple slices on a dish.

2. Drizzle or spread almond butter on each apple slice.
3. Sprinkle with ground cinnamon for an added kick of flavor.
4. Top with chopped almonds for extra crunch.

Nutrition Information (per serving):

Calories: 180 Protein: 4g Fat: 11g Carbohydrates: 20g Fiber: 5g Sugar: 14g Sodium: 2mg

Baked Sweet Potato Chips

Prep Time: 10 minutes **Cook Time:** 30 minutes **Serve:** 4 servings

Ingredients

- 2 medium sweet potatoes
- 2 tbsp olive oil
- 1/2 tsp smoked paprika
- 1/2 tsp ground turmeric
- 1/4 tsp salt
- 1/4 tsp black pepper

Instructions

1. Preheat the oven to 375° Fahrenheit (190° Celsius). Line two baking pans with parchment paper.
2. Wash and peel sweet potatoes. Using a mandoline or a sharp knife, slice them thinly to approximately 1/8-inch thickness.
3. Combine the sweet potato slices, olive oil, smoked paprika, turmeric, salt, and black pepper in a large mixing bowl.
4. Place the sweet potato slices on the prepared baking pans in a single layer, ensuring they don't overlap.
5. Bake for 25-30 minutes, flipping the slices halfway through or until the chips are crispy and lightly browned. Keep a watchful eye on the final few minutes to avoid scorching.
6. Remove from the oven and let cool completely; the chips will crisp up as they cool.

Nutrition Information (per serving):

Calories: 120 Protein: 1g Fat: 5g Carbohydrates: 18g Fiber: 3g Sugar: 4g Sodium: 100mg

Carrot Sticks with Hummus

Prep Time: 10 minutes **Cook Time:** None **Serve:** 4 servings

Ingredients

- 4 large carrots, peeled and cut into sticks
- 1 cup of hummus
- 1/2 tsp ground paprika (for garnish)
- 1/2 tsp ground turmeric

Instructions

1. Place the carrot sticks on a serving platter.
2. Place the hummus in a small bowl and season with ground paprika and turmeric if desired.
3. Serve the carrot sticks with hummus for dipping.

Nutrition Information (per serving):

Calories: 90 Protein: 2g Fat: 5g Carbohydrates: 10g Fiber: 3g Sugar: 4g Sodium: 120mg

Kale Chips with Sea Salt

Prep Time: 10 minutes **Cook Time:** 15 minutes **Serve:** 4 servings

Ingredients

- 1 bunch, kale, stems removed and leaves torn into bite-sized pieces
- 2 tbsp olive oil
- 1/2 tsp sea salt
- 1/4 tsp ground turmeric
- 1/4 tsp garlic powder (optional)

Instructions

1. Preheat the oven to 350° Fahrenheit (175° Celsius). Line a baking sheet with parchment paper.
2. Toss the kale in a large bowl with olive oil, sea salt, turmeric, and garlic powder. Toss the kale until it is uniformly covered.
3. Arrange the kale in a single layer on the prepared baking sheet, taking care not to overcrowd.

4. Bake 10-15 minutes in a preheated oven until the edges are crispy but not charred. Keep a tight check on them in the last few minutes to prevent scorching.
5. Remove from the oven and allow the kale chips to cool for a few minutes before serving.

Nutrition Information (per serving):

Calories: 70 Protein: 2g Fat: 5g Carbohydrates: 5g Fiber: 2g Sugar: 0g Sodium: 150mg

Cucumber Slices with Guacamole

Prep Time: 10 minutes **Cook Time:** None **Serve:** 4 servings

Ingredients

- 2 medium cucumbers, sliced
- 2 ripe avocados
- 1 small tomato, finely chopped
- 1/4 small red onion, finely chopped
- 1 garlic clove, minced
- Juice of 1 lime
- 1/4 tsp ground cumin
- 1/4 tsp black pepper
- 1/4 tsp salt
- 1 tbsp fresh cilantro, chopped (optional)

Instructions:

1. To make the guacamole, scrape the avocado flesh into a medium bowl and mash it with a fork until smooth.
2. Combine the diced tomato, red onion, minced garlic, lime juice, ground cumin, black pepper, and salt. Mix until well mixed. If desired, add some chopped cilantro.
3. Place the cucumber slices on a serving platter and serve with guacamole on the side for dipping.

Nutrition Information (per serving):

Calories: 130 Protein: 2g Fat: 11g Carbohydrates: 8g Fiber: 5g Sugar: 2g Sodium: 120mg

Roasted Pumpkin Seeds

Prep Time: 10 minutes

Cook Time: 25 minutes

Serve: 4 servings

Ingredients

- 1 cup of raw pumpkin seeds
- 1 tbsp olive oil
- 1/2 tsp sea salt
- 1/2 tsp smoked paprika
- 1/2 tsp ground turmeric
- 1/4 tsp black pepper

Instructions

1. Preheat the oven to 350° Fahrenheit (175° Celsius). Line a baking sheet with parchment paper.
2. Mix the cleaned and dried pumpkin seeds, olive oil, sea salt, smoked paprika, turmeric, and black pepper in a bowl. Toss the seeds until uniformly coated.
3. Place the seasoned pumpkin seeds in a single layer on the prepared baking sheet.
4. Roast the seeds in a preheated oven for 20-25 minutes, stirring halfway through, until golden and crispy.
5. Allow the roasted pumpkin seeds to cool fully before serving.

Nutrition Information (per serving):

Calories: 90 Protein: 4g Fat: 7g Carbohydrates: 3g Sugar: 0g

Turmeric Spiced Popcorn

Prep Time: 5 minutes

Cook Time: 10 minutes

Serve: 4 servings

Ingredients

- 1/2 cup of popcorn kernels
- 2 tbsp olive oil (divided)
- 1/2 tsp ground turmeric
- 1/2 tsp smoked paprika
- 1/4 tsp garlic powder (optional)
- 1/4 tsp sea salt
- 1/4 tsp black pepper

Instructions

1. In a large pot, heat 1 tablespoon olive oil over medium heat. Add the popcorn kernels and cover with the lid.
2. Cook until all kernels have popped, approximately 5-7 minutes, and shake the pot regularly to avoid burning.
3. When the popping slows, take the pot from the heat and transfer the popcorn to a large bowl.
4. In a small mixing bowl, combine the remaining tablespoon of olive oil, turmeric, smoked paprika, garlic powder (if using), sea salt, and black pepper.
5. Drizzle the spice mixture over the popcorn and toss to coat.
6. Serve immediately and enjoy!

Nutrition Information (per serving):

Calories: 110 Protein: 2g Fat: 7g Carbohydrates: 11g Fiber: 3g Sugar: 0g Sodium: 120mg

CHAPTER 8: DESSERTS

Coconut Mango Chia Pudding

Prep Time: 10 minutes

Cook Time: None

Serve: 4 servings

Ingredients:

- 1 can (13.5 oz) coconut milk
- 1/2 cup of chia seeds
- 1 tbsp maple syrup
- 1/2 tsp ground turmeric
- 1/2 tsp vanilla extract
- 1 ripe mango, peeled and diced
- Fresh mint leaves for garnish (optional)

Instructions:

1. In a medium mixing bowl, blend the coconut milk, chia seeds, maple syrup (if using), turmeric, and vanilla extract until well combined.
2. Cover the bowl and chill for at least 4 hours, preferably overnight, to let the chia seeds absorb the liquid and develop a pudding-like texture.
3. Before serving, mix the chia pudding to make a uniform texture.
4. Spoon the chia pudding into serving dishes and top with chopped mango.
5. If preferred, garnish with fresh mint leaves. Serve cold.

Nutrition Information (per serving):

Calories: 210 Protein: 3g Fat: 17g Carbohydrates: 16g Fiber: 6g Sugar: 8g Sodium: 15mg

Avocado Chocolate Mousse

Prep Time: 10 minutes

Cook Time: None

Serve: 4 servings

Ingredients

- 2 ripe avocados
- 1/4 cup of unsweetened cocoa powder
- 1/4 cup of maple syrup (or honey)
- 1/4 cup of unsweetened almond milk
- 1 tsp vanilla extract
- 1/4 tsp ground cinnamon (optional)
- Pinch of salt
- Fresh berries for garnish (optional)

Instructions:

1. Cut the avocados in half, remove the pits, and scoop out the flesh into a food processor or blender.
2. Combine the cocoa powder, maple syrup, almond milk, vanilla extract, cinnamon (if using), and a bit of salt in the blender.
3. Blend until the mixture is smooth and creamy, scraping the sides as necessary.
4. Spoon the mousse into serving dishes or glasses and chill for 30 minutes.
5. Garnish with fresh berries before serving.

Nutrition Information (per serving):

Calories: 180 Protein: 3g Fat: 14g Carbohydrates: 19g Fiber: 7g Sugar: 10g Sodium: 20mg

Baked Cinnamon Apples with Walnuts

Prep Time: 10 minutes

Cook Time: 25 minutes

Serve: 4 servings

Ingredients

- 4 medium apples cored and sliced
- 2 tbsp maple syrup
- 1 tsp ground cinnamon
- 1/4 tsp ground turmeric
- 1/4 cup of chopped walnuts
- 1 tbsp melted coconut oil
- 1/4 tsp ground nutmeg (optional)

Instructions

1. Preheat the oven to 350° Fahrenheit (175° Celsius). Lightly coat a baking dish with coconut oil.
2. Mix the apple slices, maple syrup, ground cinnamon, turmeric (if using), melted coconut oil, and nutmeg in a large bowl. Mix the apples until they are uniformly covered.
3. Spread the apple mixture in the baking dish and top with chopped walnuts.
4. Bake in the oven for 20-25 minutes or until the apples are soft and faintly caramelized.
5. Let it cool for a few minutes before serving.

Nutrition Information (per serving):

Calories: 160 Protein: 1g Fat: 7g Carbohydrates: 26g Fiber: 5g Sugar: 18g Sodium: 2mg

Almond Flour Brownies

Prep Time: 15 minutes

Cook Time: 25 minutes

Serve: 9 servings

Ingredients

- 1 cup of almond flour
- 1/4 cup of unsweetened cocoa powder
- 1/2 tsp baking powder
- 1/4 tsp salt
- 1/4 cup of coconut oil, melted
- 1/4 cup of maple syrup (or honey)
- 1/4 cup of unsweetened almond milk
- 2 tsp vanilla extract
- 1/4 cup of dark chocolate chips (optional)

Instructions

1. Preheat the oven to 350° Fahrenheit (175° Celsius). Line an 8-by-8-inch baking dish with parchment paper.
2. Combine the almond flour, cocoa powder, baking powder, and salt
3. in a large bowl.
4. Whisk together the melted coconut oil, maple syrup, almond milk, and vanilla extract in a separate bowl.
5. Pour the wet ingredients into the dry and mix until smooth. Fold in the dark chocolate chips, if desired.
6. Pour the batter into the prepared baking dish and distribute evenly.
7. Bake for 20 to 25 minutes or until a toothpick inserted in the middle comes out mostly clean.
8. Let the brownies cool fully before cutting them into squares.

Nutrition Information (per serving):

Calories: 180 Protein: 3g Fat: 14g Carbohydrates: 11g Fiber: 3g Sugar: 7g Sodium: 60mg

Blueberry Chia Pudding

Prep Time: 10 minutes (plus 4 hours chilling)

Cook Time: None

Serve: 4 servings

Ingredients

- 1 1/2 cups of unsweetened almond milk
- 1/2 cup of chia seeds
- 2 tbsp maple syrup (optional for sweetness)
- 1/2 tsp vanilla extract
- 1 cup of fresh blueberries
- 1/4 tsp ground turmeric

Instructions

1. In a medium mixing bowl, blend the almond milk, chia seeds, maple syrup (if using), vanilla extract, and turmeric until thoroughly combined.
2. Mix in 1 cup of fresh blueberries.
3. Cover the dish and chill for at least 4 hours, preferably overnight, to let the chia seeds absorb the liquid and develop a pudding-like texture.
4. Before serving, mix the chia pudding well. Spoon into serving dishes and top with more fresh blueberries.

Nutrition Information (per serving):

Calories: 150 Protein: 4g Fat: 8g Carbohydrates: 18g Fiber: 8g Sugar: 7g Sodium: 60mg

Turmeric Spiced Banana Bread

Prep Time: 15 minutes **Cook Time:** 50 minutes **Serve:** 10 servings

Ingredients

- 3 ripe bananas, mashed
- 2 large eggs
- 1/4 cup of maple syrup (or honey)
- 1/4 cup of melted coconut oil
- 1 tsp vanilla extract
- 1 1/2 cups of almond flour
- 1/2 cup of oat flour
- 1 tsp baking powder
- 1/2 tsp baking soda
- 1 tsp ground turmeric
- 1 tsp ground cinnamon
- 1/4 tsp ground nutmeg
- 1/4 tsp salt
- 1/4 cup of chopped walnuts (optional)

Instructions:

1. Preheat the oven to 350°F (175° C). Grease a 9x5-inch loaf pan or line with parchment paper.
2. In a large mixing bowl, combine the mashed bananas, eggs, maple syrup, melted coconut oil, and vanilla extract until well combined.
3. Mix the almond flour, oat flour, baking powder, baking soda, turmeric, cinnamon, nutmeg, and salt in a separate bowl.
4. Combine the dry ingredients with the wet ingredients and whisk until just combined. If desired, add the chopped walnuts.
5. Pour the batter into the prepared loaf pan and level the top.
6. Bake 45-50 minutes in a preheated oven or until a toothpick inserted in the middle comes out clean.
7. Allow the banana bread to cool in the pan for ten minutes before moving it to a wire rack to finish cooling.

Nutrition Information (per serving):

Calories: 180 Protein: 4g Fat: 10g Carbohydrates: 19g Fiber: 3g Sugar: 8g Sodium: 120mg

Dark Chocolate Avocado Truffles

Prep Time: 15 minutes (plus 1 hour chilling)

Cook Time: None

Serve: 12 truffles

Ingredients

- 1 ripe avocado, mashed
- 1 cup of dark chocolate chips (70% cocoa or higher)
- 1 tsp vanilla extract
- 1/4 cup of unsweetened cocoa powder (for rolling)
- 1/4 tsp ground cinnamon (optional)
- Pinch of salt

Instructions:

1. Melt the dark chocolate chips in a heatproof bowl over a saucepan of boiling water (double boiler technique) or in a microwave in 20-second increments until smooth, stirring occasionally.
2. In a medium bowl, mash the avocado until smooth and creamy. Stir in the melted chocolate, vanilla essence, cinnamon (if using), and salt until well blended.
3. Cover the bowl and chill for about 1 hour or until the mixture is stiff enough to scoop.
4. After chilling, use a spoon to scoop parts of the dough and shape them into 1-inch balls.
5. Roll each truffle in the unsweetened cocoa powder until well-covered.
6. Put the truffles on a platter and refrigerate until ready to serve.

Nutrition Information (per truffle):

Calories: 70 Protein: 1g Fat: 5g Carbohydrates: 6g Sugar: 3g Sodium: 5mg

Almond Butter Chocolate Chip Cookies

Prep Time: 10 minutes **Cook Time:** 12 minutes **Serve:** 12 cookies

Ingredients

- 1 cup of almond butter (unsweetened)
- 1/3 cup of maple syrup or honey
- 1 large egg
- 1/2 tsp baking soda
- 1/2 tsp vanilla extract
- 1/4 tsp ground cinnamon (optional)
- 1/4 cup of dark chocolate chips
- Pinch of salt

Instructions

1. Preheat the oven to 350°F (175° C). Line a baking sheet with parchment paper.
2. In a large mixing bowl, add almond butter, maple syrup (or honey), egg (or flax egg), baking soda, vanilla extract, cinnamon (if using), and a sprinkle of salt. Mix until well mixed.
3. Fold in the dark chocolate chips.
4. Scoop out tablespoons of dough and shape into balls. Place them on the prepared baking sheet, approximately 2 inches apart.
5. Gently press your fingers down on each dough ball to flatten it slightly.
6. Bake in a preheated oven for 10-12 minutes or until the sides brown.
7. Allow the cookies to cool on the baking sheet for 5 minutes before moving them to a wire rack to finish cooling.

Nutrition Information (per cookie):

Calories: 120 Protein: 3g Fat: 8g Fiber: 2g Sugar: 6g Sodium: 45mg

Lemon Coconut Energy Balls

Prep Time: 10 minutes

Cook Time: None

Serve: 12 energy balls

Ingredients

- 1 cup of rolled oats
- 1/2 cup of unsweetened shredded coconut (plus extra for rolling)
- 1/4 cup of almond butter
- 1/4 cup of honey or maple syrup
- Zest of 1 lemon
- Juice of 1 lemon
- 1/2 tsp vanilla extract
- Pinch of salt

Instructions:

1. Combine the rolled oats, coconut flakes, almond butter, honey (or maple syrup), lemon zest, lemon juice, vanilla essence, and salt in a large mixing bowl. Mix until everything is fully combined and produces a sticky consistency.
2. Scoop out tablespoon-sized amounts of the mixture and form into balls.
3. Roll each energy ball in more crushed coconut to cover the exterior.
4. Put the energy balls in an airtight jar and chill for at least 30 minutes before serving.

Nutrition Information (per energy ball):

Calories: 80 Protein: 2g Fat: 4g Carbohydrates: 10g Fiber: 2g Sugar: 5g Sodium: 10mg

Banana Almond Oat Bars

Prep Time: 10 minutes

Cook Time: 25 minutes

Serve: 12 bars

Ingredients

- 2 ripe bananas, mashed
- 1 1/2 cups of rolled oats
- 1/2 cup of almond butter
- 1/4 cup of honey or maple syrup
- 1/2 tsp vanilla extract
- 1/2 tsp ground cinnamon
- 1/4 tsp ground turmeric (optional, for anti-inflammatory benefits)
- 1/4 cup of chopped almonds
- 1/4 cup of dark chocolate chips (optional)

Instructions:

1. Preheat the oven to 350°F (175° C). Line an 8-by-8-inch baking dish with parchment paper.
2. Add the mashed bananas, almond butter, honey (or maple syrup), and vanilla extract in a large bowl. Mix well until smooth.
3. Combine the rolled oats, cinnamon, turmeric (if using), and chopped almonds with the wet mixture. Stir until everything is well combined.
4. Fold in the dark chocolate chips, if desired.
5. Pour the mixture into the prepared baking dish and distribute evenly.
6. Bake in a preheated oven for 20-25 minutes or until the sides are brown and the middle is firm.
7. Allow the bars to cool fully in the pan before cutting into twelve squares.

Nutrition Information (per bar):

Calories: 130 Protein: 3g Fat: 7g Carbohydrates: 15g Fiber: 3g Sugar: 6g Sodium: 10mg

30 DAYS MEAL PLAN

Day	Breakfast	Lunch	Dinner	Snack/Dessert
01	Quinoa Breakfast Bowl with Blueberries	Mediterranean Chickpea Salad	Grilled Chicken with Turmeric and Lime	Almond Butter and Banana Bites
02	Sweet Potato and Avocado Toast	Roasted Brussels Sprouts with Balsamic Glaze	Baked Salmon with Dill and Lemon	Coconut Mango Chia Pudding
03	Oatmeal with Almonds and Flaxseeds	Roasted Beet and Goat Cheese Salad	Vegan Lentil and Spinach Curry	Baked Sweet Potato Chips
04	Chia Seed Pudding with Mixed Berries	Grilled Asparagus with Lemon	Garlic Shrimp with Zucchini Noodles	Avocado Chocolate Mousse
05	Turmeric and Spinach Scrambled Eggs	Cucumber and Dill Salad	Baked Chicken Breasts with Lemon and Herbs	Carrot Sticks with Hummus
06	Vegan Banana Pancakes	Mixed Berry and Spinach Salad	Lemon Herb Grilled Mackerel	Peanut Butter and Dark Chocolate Bites
07	Ginger Pear Smoothie Bowl	Spicy Black Bean Soup	Grilled Turkey Burgers with Avocado	Roasted Pumpkin Seeds
08	Coconut Yogurt with Turmeric Granola	Quinoa and Roasted Beet Salad	Garlic Shrimp with Zucchini Noodles	Flourless Almond Butter Brownies
09	Sweet Potato and Kale Hash	Vegan Cauliflower Tacos	Roasted Chicken with Garlic and Thyme	Baked Cinnamon Apples with Walnuts
10	Avocado and Egg Breakfast Wrap	Tomato and White Bean Soup	Seared Scallops with Cauliflower Puree	Mixed Berry Parfait with Coconut Yogurt
11	Almond Butter Toast with Chia Seeds	Roasted Butternut Squash with Pecans	Chicken and Sweet Potato Stir-Fry	Roasted Chickpeas with Paprika
12	Green Smoothie with Kale and Pineapple	Broccoli and Cranberry Salad	Moroccan Vegetable Tagine	Lemon Coconut Energy Balls
13	Almond Butter and Banana Toast	Pea and Mint Soup	Grilled Tuna with Avocado Salsa	Baked Zucchini Chips
14	Vegan Eggplant Parmesan	Grilled Portobello Mushrooms with Garlic	Coconut Curry Salmon	Dark Chocolate Avocado Truffles
15	Berry Almond Overnight Oats	Zesty Lemon Broccoli	Chicken Stir-Fry with Bell Peppers	Carrot and Apple Slaw
16	Vegan Stuffed Peppers with Quinoa	Broccoli and Almond Soup	Grilled Chicken Skewers with Veggies	Chia Pudding with Almond Butter

17	Spinach and Feta Omelette	Cucumber Slices with Guacamole	Balsamic Glazed Chicken Thighs	Roasted Sweet Potatoes with Turmeric
18	Quinoa and Berry Breakfast Cups	Mixed Berry and Spinach Salad	Pesto-Crusted Halibut	Almond Flour Brownies
19	Zucchini Bread with Walnuts	Chicken Noodle Soup with Turmeric	Vegan Lentil and Spinach Curry	Ginger Spiced Carrot Cake
20	Coconut Yogurt Parfait with Granola	Grilled Asparagus with Lemon	Garlic Parmesan Crusted Cod	Spicy Roasted Almonds
21	Turmeric Oatmeal with Blueberries	Quinoa and Black Bean Salad	Herb-Crusted Lamb Chops	Raspberry Coconut Bliss Balls
22	Almond Butter Toast with Banana	Spiced Lentil and Carrot Patties	Grilled Shrimp with Pineapple Salsa	Frozen Yogurt Bark with Berries
23	Vegan Eggplant Parmesan	Sweet Potato and Ginger Soup	Grilled Lamb with Mint Sauce	Dark Chocolate Dipped Strawberries
24	Vegan Vegetable Paella	Carrot and Coriander Soup	Lemon Garlic Butter Shrimp	Coconut Almond Date Squares
25	Sweet Potato and Avocado Toast	Roasted Vegetable Quinoa Bowl	Turkey and Spinach Meatballs	Almond and Date Energy Balls
26	Turmeric Spiced Banana Bread	Vegan Chickpea Salad Wrap	Slow-Cooked Beef and Sweet Potato Stew	Banana Almond Oat Bars
27	Avocado and Egg Breakfast Wrap	Roasted Beet and Goat Cheese Salad	Fish Tacos with Mango Salsa	Vegan Lemon Bars with Coconut Crust
28	Chia Seed Chocolate Pudding	Roasted Carrots with Honey and Ginger	Baked Snapper with Turmeric and Ginger	Coconut Macaroons with Dark Chocolate
29	Vegan Pumpkin Pie with Almond Crust	Steamed Green Beans with Almonds	Chicken Tenders with Almond Flour Crust	Flaxseed Crackers with Avocado Spread
30	Turmeric Oatmeal with Almonds	Cauliflower Rice with Herbs	Shrimp and Broccoli Stir-Fry	Coconut and Date Bliss Balls

Printed in Dunstable, United Kingdom